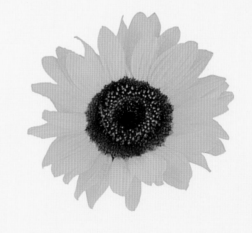

NATURAL
BEAUTY

NATURAL BEAUTY

MAKING AND USING PURE AND SIMPLE BEAUTY PRODUCTS

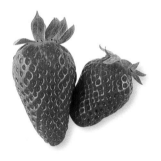

GAIL DUFF

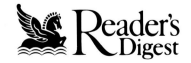

THE READER'S DIGEST ASSOCIATION, INC.
Pleasantville, New York/Montreal

A READER'S DIGEST BOOK

Conceived and produced by Breslich & Foss Ltd.

Edited by Janet Ravenscroft
Designed by Roger Daniels
Illustrations by Lynette Conway

Volume copyright © 1998 by Breslich & Foss Ltd
Text copyright © 1998 by Gail Duff

Library of Congress Cataloging in Publication Data

Duff, Gail.
    Natural beauty : making and using pure and simple beauty products / Gail Duff.
    Includes index.
    ISBN 0-7621-0032-X. (pbk.) —
    ISBN 0-7621-0033-8 (hc)
    1. Cosmetics. I. Title.
TP983.D83   1998
646.7'2—dc21   97-31659

Printed in Hong Kong

CONTENTS

Foreword

Natural beauty is about feeling good on the inside so that you look good on the outside. It is about taking care of your whole being, and that means your diet and exercise program as well as your skin and hair. It is not about putting on layers of makeup, or being liberal with the hair spray, but about caring for your body so that it looks good without artificial embellishment. Of course, you can boost the effect with makeup, but it is what is there naturally that makes the real difference.

The outside of your body is like a barometer. If you are happy or sad, tired or depressed, if you have eaten badly, drank too much, or not done enough exercise it will show, so lifestyle is the thing to work on first. Then you have to take care of your outside by cleansing your body, exfoliating the skin when necessary, moisturizing, and nourishing it.

Making your own, or at least some of your own, beauty treatments is just part of this general care. Experimenting with lotions and potions is also highly rewarding and great fun. You might save a little money,

you will certainly know where your face, hair, and body preparations come from and what they contain, and you will have the satisfaction of knowing that no animal's well-being has been sacrificed for the sake of your own.

As I wrote this book, I realized that no one in this day and age is going to be able to follow every beauty routine contained within it every day: there would be no time to do anything else. Use the treatments whenever you feel you need to pamper yourself or when you feel that a part of you needs special treatment, and gradually absorb the advice about general health and diet. Set aside certain days when you can experiment with things like creams and lotions. Get to know the quick and easy treatments that can be worked into your daily routine. Keep certain things like sun protection in the back of your mind at all times. Sneak in face or hand exercises whenever you have a moment. If you come to think more about yourself, how you feel and what you need, then I think I will have succeeded.

GAIL DUFF

BEAUTY FROM THE INSIDE

"Beauty is only skin deep" is an old cliché, but there is no better way of saying that the skin reflects whatever is going on inside your body. You can cover skin with moisturizers and makeup, but without feeding it well and caring for it from the inside you can rarely be truly beautiful.

Skin protects and supports the delicate tissues and vital organs that lie just beneath the surface. Our skin breathes and excretes waste materials and provides a growing pad for hair. It is fed nutrients and oxygen by tiny blood vessels that in turn pick up their cargoes from the food we take in and the air we breathe.

Skin is made up of two layers: the outer epidermis and the inner dermis. Both are flexible and elastic to allow movement of the body without distorting the skin. The dermis is the thicker layer. It contains blood vessels that bring nourishment and a lymphatic system that drains waste. Here also are two types of stretchy fiber, known as collagen fibers, that are made of protein and elastin. Collagen fibers give the skin the "stretch-and-spring-back" quality that helps it to withstand bumps and knocks. Hairs begin their growth in the dermis, and nerve endings and hair follicles found here make the skin sensitive to touch and pain. Sweat glands in the dermis release

moisture that helps to control the body's temperature. Sebum, a natural lubricant and moisturizer, is produced in the sebaceous glands in the dermis. It mixes with sweat and forms a thin film on the skin called the acid mantle. This lends protection against infection and bacteria.

Skin cells are formed in what is called the *stratum germinativum* (the layer where growth begins). This is the lowest layer of the epidermis. The cells are continually replaced from beneath, so a new cell is gradually pushed upward toward the surface. As the cell moves upward it begins to die and, by the time it reaches the surface, it has flattened and hardened to form the *stratum corneum*. This hard, dead, insensitive layer protects the living cells beneath. Eventually, the old cells flake away from the skin and are replaced. This process is called desquamation and takes an average of twenty-one to twenty-eight days. The younger the skin, the quicker this cycle of renewal will be.

Skin is a vital, functioning part of us, yet how often is "a lifestyle for a healthy skin" mentioned? There are "healthy heart," "stress reducing," and "cancer preventive" lifestyles by the score, but skin seems to lose out.

Skin reflects the state of our bodies and our minds. Feeling run down? Then look in the mirror. Your skin will not look its sparkling best either. Have you eaten too much greasy food? Then watch those pimples appear in the more oily parts of your face. Have you been on a crash diet, eating nothing but lettuce leaves for days? Perhaps the skin on your arms or legs has gone dry and flaky. Does stress attack you in the middle of the night? Watch for the dark rings under your eyes. The better things are inside, the more naturally beautiful you will look.

GENERAL HEALTH

Health is a general state of well-being. To achieve it, take care of yourself: eat a balanced diet, drink alcohol in moderation, don't smoke, get enough sleep, try to reduce stress, and exercise as often as possible. Simple really. Sounds boring? Well, try it and see. You will probably find that the healthier you feel, the more energy you have, and a person with a lot of energy very often has a greater capacity for enjoying life. If it sounds like an impossible lifestyle, make small changes first and see how things develop.

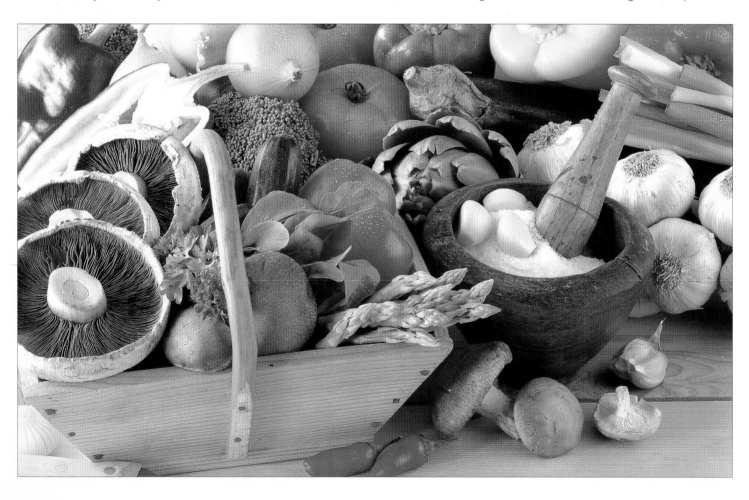

Breakfast:

Whole grain toast with honey or unsweetened jam

Poached egg on whole grain toast

Muesli or other whole grain cereal with milk or plain yogurt with chopped fruit added

Fresh chopped fruits with plain yogurt

Light meal:

Small piece of grilled or poached fish

Large mixed salad with small amount of protein-rich food

Whole grain sandwiches with salad filling

Baked potato with a little butter or low-fat spread salad

Homemade or other nourishing vegetable soup with whole grain bread

Homemade dip with vegetables

Fresh fruit for dessert

Main meal:

Small meat or vegetarian protein dish with potatoes, whole grain rice, or pasta, and at least two other vegetables

Fruit salad with plain yogurt for dessert

Snacks:

Fresh fruit

Fingers of raw vegetables

Whole grain biscuits

Plain yogurt

When you are young, you can get away with a bad diet, a hectic lifestyle, and lack of sleep, and still look great. But there will come a day when you look in the mirror and see the first gray hair or the first wrinkle. If you take extra care as early as possible, you may well be delaying the onset of those first signs of aging.

DIET

A healthy diet should provide all the nutrients a body needs: protein for bodybuilding, carbohydrates for energy, fats in moderation for lubrication, a wide selection of vitamins and minerals for the proper functioning and repair of body tissues, plus fiber to help eliminate waste.

Eating a lot of any one food, however nourishing it is, will give you plenty of one or two nutrients and none of any of the others. A variety of foods eaten every day will provide a wide range of different nutrients. Try to include some

carbohydrate foods, such as whole wheat bread, pasta, and rice; at least four servings each of fresh fruit and vegetables; protein foods such as lean meat, fish, cheese, eggs, beans, and nuts. Combine the last two with a whole grain food so you get the right kind of protein.

Some fat is necessary for good health, but you should keep the amount of animal fats you consume to a minimum. By all means have butter on your toast, but don't overdo it. Choose lean meat and cook it with sunflower or olive oil. Nuts are a good source of "healthy" fat.

The fresher and less processed a food, the more nutrients it contains. If it has been chopped, cooked, mixed with other ingredients, dried or frozen, it will not contain the same goodness it began with. For optimum health, buy fresh ingredients and cook them yourself (or eat them raw).

Sugar is a highly refined carbohydrate that brings no nutrients with it in its white form, and only a few when left brown. Too much sugar piles on the calories and also uses up essential B vitamins in its digestion. Try to cut it down.

Processing also includes the refinement of carbohydrate foods such as wheat or rice. When the whole grain of the wheat is ground to make whole meal flour, the tiny growing point (the germ), and the outer coating (the bran), are retained. The germ contains most of the nutrients. The bran provides the fiber that helps us to eliminate waste. If a body cannot eliminate waste, the skin may develop a gray, sallow look. If you eat a balanced, relatively high-fiber diet, with plenty of raw fruits and vegetables you should have no problems.

Extra bran used to be a recommended remedy, but bran alone can deplete the body's iron supplies. It is far better to eat a high-fiber cereal or whole wheat bread. High-fiber foods are also more satisfying, and prevent us from overeating. Whenever possible, therefore, choose whole grain bread, pasta, and brown rice. Other fiber-rich foods are fresh fruits and vegetables. Eat them whenever you can, as desserts, as part of a meal, and as snacks between meals. They provide a wide range of vitamins and minerals, and help ensure a healthy skin.

Water is essential for good health. It moisturizes your skin from the inside and helps waste and toxins to flush through the body. Ideally you should drink eight glasses of water a day. If you find mineral water in this quantity too expensive, drink filtered tap water. Cut down on caffeine-rich drinks such as tea or coffee, choosing herb teas instead.

Dietary enemies

Both smoking cigarettes and drinking alcohol deplete the body's vitamin supply, especially of vitamins B and C, both of which are essential for maintaining a healthy skin. Toxins from alcohol and cigarette smoke are carried around the body in the bloodstream and smoking can restrict the blood flow to the skin. Coarse, aging skin can be the result.

Many medications, such as antibiotics, can upset the skin's natural flora. This is because our skin is home to friendly bacteria that help to combat germs. Antibiotics are not choosy. They may kill off harmful bacteria, but they also kill off the ones we need, both in the digestive system and in the skin. The simple remedy, if you are on prescribed medicines, is to eat at least ⅔ cup/150 ml plain yogurt every day while the course of treatment lasts, and for two weeks thereafter.

SLEEP

Getting plenty of sleep is one of the other major contributors to maintaining healthy and glowing skin. During sleep, the body can repair itself undisturbed. It can also begin the process of ridding the tissues of toxins and waste materials. Without sleep, skin can develop a lack of tone and begin to look rather loose and baggy. Too many late nights can lead to dark rings under the eyes and premature aging of the skin.

The body naturally relaxes as you sleep. All tightness leaves the muscles and this, in turn, helps to smooth out expression-formed wrinkles in the face. Dreams, even though you may not remember them, can help you to sort out day-to-day problems, thus relieving you of stress the following day.

People differ in the amount of sleep that they need. By the time you are an adult you probably have a good idea of how much you need, even though you may not adhere to it. Average sleep needs are from six to eight hours, and the hours before midnight are the most valuable when it comes to restful sleep. The body responds best to the same pattern of sleep week by week. If possible, make certain nights late nights and others early ones. Bodies like routine, even if people don't.

In order to sleep, both your mind and body should be relaxed. Some people can just get into bed and fall asleep right away, others, for a variety of reasons, have difficulty. Try as many of the following as possible:

• Stop working. You have put in a busy day, you deserve to rest. Whether it is ironing, washing dishes, or doing office work, make a conscious decision to stop.

• You may think that watching the television or a video is one of the most relaxing things that you can do but it isn't. Turn off the television.

• Enjoy the silence or put on a relaxing tape. Don't let anyone else choose the tape for you.

• Make yourself a warm drink made from milk—which is rich in calcium and promotes sleep—or an herbal drink designed for bedtime. Avoid tea and coffee at bedtime.

• If possible, eat your main meal two hours before going to bed to allow it to digest and to get rid of any uncomfortable "full" feeling. Don't eat anything rich just before bedtime, but don't go to bed hungry. Have something like plain crackers or a small sandwich about half an hour before you retire.

• If you have to remember something the next day, write it down and leave it in a prominent place outside the bedroom. The same applies to problems. Write them down and resolve to deal with them in the morning.

• Try to resolve household arguments before going to bed. If you are angry or upset, sleep may not be easy.

• Warm baths are relaxing last thing at night. Pamper yourself. Add some relaxing, perfumed bath preparation, light a candle instead of turning on the light. Lie back and let your tension float away.

• Keep your bedroom as neat as possible so it is a special place to which you enjoy going. Light some incense or vaporize some perfumed oil, choosing relaxing scents, not the stimulating ones. Put water into the top of a vaporizer and add a few drops of essential oil. Then put a lighted teacup candle underneath. Electric vaporizers are also available.

• Choose candlelight instead of electric light. (Make sure to blow out the candles before falling asleep.)

• Make love with your partner. This may well keep you awake longer than you intended, but sleep is always quick to come and very deep afterwards.

EXERCISE

Exercise is important because it brings extra oxygen into your system and increases blood circulation. This means there is a greater turnaround of nutrients and waste products in every organ of your body, including your skin and hair. Keeping your system cleansed and vital helps you feel and look good.

There are two types of exercise. One is active, such as a workout in the gym or a set of aerobic exercises. The other is more passive, such as yoga or other forms of stretching exercise, and concentrates on the body's suppleness. In an ideal world we would include each in our regular routine.

Aerobic exercise should make you slightly out of breath, but not leave you breathless and exhausted. You should exercise at least twenty minutes three times a week, preceded by warm-up exercises and finished with a cool-down. Small, regular periods of exercise are far more efficient in toning the body than indulging in a long period of frantic movement once a week.

If you are deskbound at work, try to get up and walk about once every hour to stretch your limbs, and do a short series of stretching exercises daily. A daily, brisk, twenty-minute walk is a perfect first stage to fitness.

There are many forms of exercise programs available and the important thing is that you should choose the one that suits you best. Consider your physical abilities, age, and the facilities available within your locality. Never rush into an exercise program or go for the advanced exercises first. Start with gentle exercises and gradually work up to a routine that your body can cope with. If you have not taken part in any regular exercise for some time it is also a good idea to get a physical from your regular doctor. No matter what your age, if your program is a sensible one, you will always improve with time.

HEALTHY MIND—HEALTHY BODY

Any mental stress will manifest itself within your body and show in your outward appearance. Many people, for example, acknowledge that they have a "weak point" which is affected as soon as they experience stress. One person may develop a sore throat, another a headache, another an aching limb, all the result of some stressful occurrence. It is really nature's way of telling you that you have had enough and you should take time out. If you develop an ailment you have to stop and nurse yourself until you feel better. It is this resting time that your mind needs.

Stress is a natural function. The release of adrenaline into the bloodstream prepares us for "fight or flight." When we are in a dangerous situation or when suffering from shock, adrenaline helps us to cope. What is not productive is continual stress that takes a hold and will not go away.

The aim, then, is to reduce stress. When under stress you may feel alone and that no one can help you. Lesson number one is to care for yourself. Allow yourself the time to do something that makes you feel good. Go for a walk and look at the things around you.

Learning to relax

There are many relaxation techniques around, and you can go to classes to learn them. Here is one that might help. Lie down on your back somewhere comfortable and warm, but not too hot. Close your eyes. Stretch all your limbs together and gradually let go. Do this twice. Imagine you are somewhere that you have enjoyed being such as a beach or a grassy bank. Imagine the sun above you. Imagine its rays touching your body and warming you through. Think about your feet. Flex them and relax them. Do the same

with your lower legs, then the top of your legs, and gradually work your way up your body to the top of your head. Feel yourself to be weightless and imagine the golden glow of the sun penetrating your body. Apart from this, try to keep your mind blank. Lie there for as long as you can. When you want to finish, consciously feel each part of your body, from the toes up, keeping it relaxed but being aware of it. Imagine the room that you are in and think of the floor or the earth beneath your feet. Slowly open your eyes.

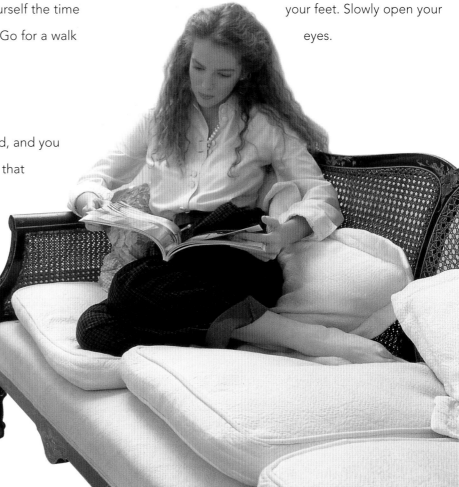

MAKING YOUR OWN BEAUTY PREPARATIONS

Making your own beauty treatments is not difficult, and you don't need a complicated range of equipment or ingredients. Many of the things you need can be found in the utensils and ingredients cupboards of the average, well-stocked kitchen, and the rest are easily bought.

What you cannot obtain are the chemical ingredients that are often to be found in even the most natural of store-bought preparations. Nor do you have access to the whipping, stirring, and mixing machinery that is used in most commercial manufacture. This means that the texture of your homemade creams may vary from bought ones, but this does not make them any less efficient or less of a joy to use. You can't expect them to be exactly the same, just as a homemade loaf of bread is rarely of a similar texture to a store-bought one.

Before starting to make your own cosmetics, you must prepare a working area in your kitchen. As with cooking, you need some basic equipment, hot and cold running water, an electric outlet, and a stove. Give yourself plenty of room to work, and clear the area of all food before you start mixing.

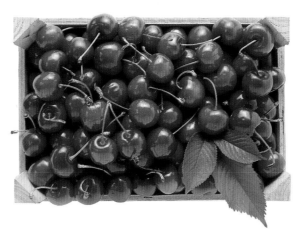

When making a recipe, have all the ingredients prepared (chopped, grated, etc.) and laid out on a table. Similarly, have all the necessary equipment ready before you begin.

EQUIPMENT

Opposite is a list of the equipment you will need to make the recipes in this book—you won't require every item for every single recipe. When starting to make your own cosmetics, use your regular kitchen equipment. If you decide that it is to become a regular hobby, consider keeping a separate set of basic equipment. This will avoid getting beeswax in the soup!

All your equipment should be clean before you begin, and your jars, containers, and bottles sterilized. Even though they look clean, they may be harboring a thin film of dust or dirt that could contaminate your new cosmetics, or make them get moldy.

To sterilize plastic containers, first make sure they are heat-resistant. Place them in a saucepan, cover with water, and bring gently to a boil. Lift them out with tongs and let them drain. Dry with a clean cloth.

Glass containers can be sterilized in a low oven, about 100°F (40°C). Wash them first and place them on their side on the oven racks. Leave them for ten minutes. All lids and tops should be sterilized as well. Both metal and plastic containers can be treated in the same way as plastic ones. **Important** To prevent contamination from condensation, always allow the recipe you are making to cool completely before sealing it into its container.

USING HERBS

The most commonly used herbs are listed in the chart on page 19. Others are given in specific sections and recipes. Some dried herbs, such as chamomile and peppermint, can be bought from supermarkets in the form of herbal teas. More unusual ones, such as nettle or comfrey, must be bought from herbalists or health food stores. Herbs are most frequently made into infusions and decoctions, and recipes for these are given throughout the book.

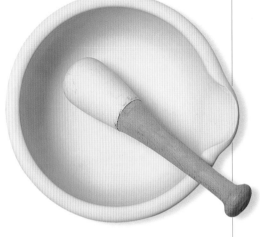

EQUIPMENT YOU WILL NEED

- A selection of easily washable bowls of varying sizes, the smaller and medium-sized ones to be heat-resistant
- Heat-resistant measuring pitchers
- Stainless steel or enamel saucepans
- Double boiler or a saucepan large enough to hold a medium-sized bowl standing on a trivet
- Tea kettle
- Scales
- Measuring spoons
- Selection of wooden spoons of varying sizes
- Metal teaspoon and tablespoon
- Mortar and pestle
- Coffee grinder
- Food processor or blender
- Sterilized jars, pots, and bottles in which to store finished products
- Large, plastic dishwashing pan

CIDER VINEGAR

Cider vinegar is produced by fermenting natural apple juice. It is a rich source of potassium and contains significant amounts of phosphorus, sodium, magnesium, calcium, iron, fluorine, and chlorine. Added to bath water, it both softens and helps to restore the natural acid balance of the skin.

INGREDIENTS

For the main ingredients that are used for skin care, refer to the chart on pages 20-21. Do not buy all the ingredients at once. Decide which recipes you would like to make, and which ingredients are suitable for your skin type. Everybody's skin is different and reacts differently to certain ingredients and preparations. Before you go ahead and make a beauty treatment, do a "patch test" to check whether you are allergic to any of the ingredients. The simplest way of doing this is to rub a little of the ingredient onto a part of your skin that is delicate but which does not show, such as the inside of your arm. Leave it for 12 hours.

If you have any sort of allergic reaction, do not use that particular ingredient. To check the effect of a herb, make up an infusion following the instructions on page 17, and dab it on to your skin in the same way.

A range of vegetable and nut oils is used in the book. Some, such as olive, coconut, or sunflower, can be bought as foods. The rest can be bought from herbalists, health food shops, pharmacists, drugstores, and suppliers of essential oils for aromatherapy.

It is important to buy reputable brands of essential oils from aromatherapy suppliers or health food stores. In most cases, the more expensive the oils are, the better the quality, but it is worth getting advice from other users. There is more information on this topic on pages 98-99.

Other ingredients in the recipes that might be slightly less familiar include:

DECOCTION

Decoctions are usually greater in strength than infusions. The herb is put into a saucepan with cold water, brought to a boil and simmered for a given time. The liquid can be left to stand for a time after simmering, or it can be immediately strained off. The amount of herb, the simmering time, and the standing time can all affect strength. An average strength decoction is made by simmering 1 tbsp fresh chopped herb or 1 tsp dried in 1¼ cups/275 ml water for ten minutes. It can then be strained immediately or left, covered, for ten minutes before straining.

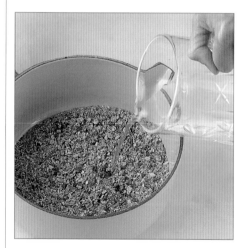

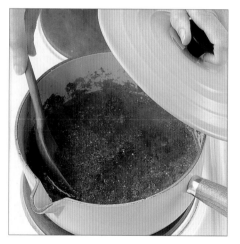

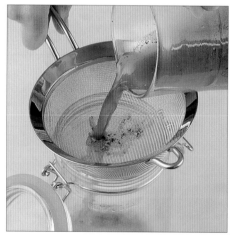

1 Fresh or dried herbs are placed in a stainless steel saucepan and covered with cold water.

2 The mixture is brought to the boil, then simmered.

3 The decoction is strained into a clean container ready for use.

• *Arrowroot*: This is a white powder obtained by grinding the dried roots of the arrowroot plant. It is used to thicken sauces and other liquids, in a similar way to corn flour. It is used in teeth and hair preparations.

• *Beeswax*: This is the wax used by bees to make honey cells in the hive. Beeswax for cosmetic use has usually been purified by melting and straining. It is available in blocks, disks or sheets in its natural yellow color or as disks in a more purified white form. It can be obtained from honey producers, candle makers' suppliers, and herbalists.

• *Borax*: Also known as sodium borate, borax is available as fine white crystals. It is added to washing water for its softening properties. Used very sparingly in beauty preparations, it will help to amalgamate the other ingredients.

• *Cocoa butter*: This is obtained by roasting and then grinding cacao beans and then separating out the fat. Chocolate is what remains after the process. The pure "butter" is sold in blocks. It is similar in texture to soap, but melts easily at a temperature of about 100°F (40°C).

INFUSION

Making an infusion is the same as making a cup of tea. An amount of the dried or fresh chopped herb is put into a container and boiling water is poured on it. The mixture is covered, brewed for a while, and then strained. Amounts and times are given in most recipes. The more herb that is used to a given amount of water and the longer it is left, the stronger the infusion. An average strength infusion is made with 1 tbsp fresh chopped herb or 1 tsp dried to 1 cup/250 ml water.

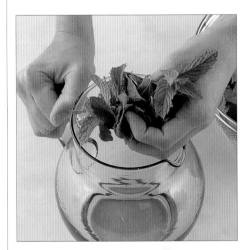

1 Fresh or dried herbs are placed in a heat-proof container.

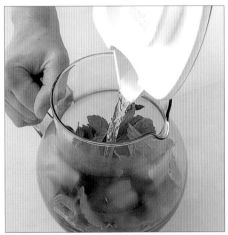

2 Boiling water is poured onto the herbs, and the mixture covered and left to infuse.

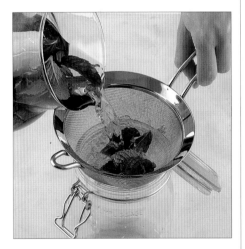

3 The cooled infusion is strained into a clean container ready for use.

Cocoa butter is available from herbalists and drugstores.

• *Cultured buttermilk:* Buttermilk was originally the name given to the whey left in the churn after the butter had been made. Now it is the name for milk to which an acid culture has been added. Unlike yogurt, it retains its liquid nature. If it is unavailable, use a thin, plain yogurt for the recipes.

• *Fuller's earth:* This is a type of clay used in the textile industry for fulling (softening) cloth, that comes in the form of a fine, gray powder. It is available from herbalists and mail-order sources, and is perfectly harmless when used on the skin or hair. It acts as a carrier for other ingredients.

• *Glycerine:* This is a vegetable product, available as a clear, slightly thickened liquid. It is a natural moisturizer which helps to draw moisture from the lower skin area to the surface.

• *Kaolin powder:* This fine white powdered clay is used for making porcelain and can be found at ceramic supply stores. It has neutral properties and can be used as a carrier for other ingredients.

• *Lanolin:* The natural oil from sheep's wool. It is similar in composition to sebum, the natural oil on human skin. It has an emollient effect and also helps the skin to retain moisture. Lanolin is usually bought from drugstores in the form of a rich, yellow-colored, sticky cream.

• *Rosewater/orange flower water:* These fragrant waters are the byproducts of the manufacture of the essential oils that come from rose and orange flowers. In the process, petals are subjected to concentrated steam which releases the essential oils. When the steam condenses, oil and water are separated. Rose and orange flower water are delicately scented and make natural skin moisturizers.

• *Tincture of benzoin:* Benzoin is a resin that comes from the benzoin tree (*Styrax benzoin*). It is used in aromatic preparations, such as potpourris, as a fixative. A tincture is made by steeping it in alcohol. Used in beauty preparations, it has a tautening effect. Tincture of benzoin can be bought from drugstores and herbalists.

• *White petroleum jelly:* This is often marketed under the tradename Vaseline. It is a translucent solid mixture of hydrocarbons, and is well-known for the soothing and softening effects it has on the skin.

• *Witch hazel:* Distilled witch hazel is a clear lotion produced from the twigs and bark of the witch hazel tree. It tones the skin, helping to close the pores. Witch hazel is a Native American healing herb which was adopted by early settlers and eventually taken to Europe.

Many different herbs are used in the recipes. If one is unavailable, you can often find an equally good substitute. This chart is intended as a guide to choosing the right herbs for your needs. As a general rule, oily skin needs astringent herbs that tauten and promote the closing of pores. Dry and mature skins need emollient herbs that will supplement the skin's own protective oils. All of these herbs soften, soothe and lubricate.

| HERB | Anti-inflammatory | Antiseptic | Astringent | Cleansing | Emollient | Invigorating | Moisturizing | Soothing | Toning | SKIN TYPE | | |
										Normal	Oily	Dry/Mature
Chamomile	❑			❑				❑	❑	❑	❑	❑
Comfrey					❑		❑	❑	❑	❑	❑	
Elderflower			❑	❑			❑	❑	❑	❑	❑	❑
Fennel			❑	❑				❑	❑	❑	❑	
Lady's mantle					❑			❑	❑	❑		❑
Lavender		❑				❑		❑	❑	❑	❑	
Lemon balm								❑	❑	❑	❑	
Linden flowers				❑	❑		❑	❑	❑	❑		
Marigold			❑	❑			❑	❑	❑	❑	❑	❑
Marshmallow					❑			❑	❑	❑	❑	❑
Mint			❑					❑	❑		❑	
Nettle				❑		❑		❑	❑	❑	❑	❑
Parsley				❑				❑	❑	❑	❑	
Rosemary						❑		❑	❑	❑	❑	
Sage		❑	❑					❑	❑	❑	❑	
Thyme		❑		❑		❑		❑	❑	❑	❑	
Violet				❑	❑			❑	❑	❑	❑	
Witch hazel			❑					❑	❑	❑	❑	
Woodruff								❑	❑	❑	❑	
Yarrow			❑					❑	❑	❑	❑	

The food ingredients used for skin care preparations are easy to obtain. Most can be found in supermarkets and stores. Others, such as brewer's yeast or bran, can be bought in health food stores. An ingredient under the heading + Acid is one that helps to restore the acid balance of the skin. Suncare covers pre- and aftersun treatments.

	Cleansing	Exfoliant	Toning	Moisturizing	+ Acid	Softening	Suncare	SKIN TYPE Normal	Oily	Dry/Mature
Almond, ground	✓	✓	✓	✓		✓	✓	✓	✓	✓
Almond oil	✓			✓		✓	✓	✓		✓
Apricot			✓			✓	✓	✓	✓	✓
Apricot oil	✓			✓		✓	✓	✓		✓
Avocado	✓			✓		✓	✓	✓	✓	✓
Avocado oil	✓			✓		✓	✓	✓		✓
Banana						✓	✓	✓		✓
Barley	✓	✓		✓		✓		✓	✓	✓
Beeswax	✓	✓		✓		✓	✓	✓	✓	✓
Benzoin	✓							✓	✓	
Borax	✓					✓		✓	✓	✓
Bran		✓				✓		✓	✓	
Butter				✓		✓	✓	✓		✓
Buttermilk	✓	✓		✓	✓	✓	✓	✓	✓	
Cocoa butter	✓			✓		✓	✓	✓	✓	✓
Cornmeal	✓	✓	✓	✓		✓		✓	✓	✓
Cream, fresh				✓		✓	✓	✓		✓
Cream, sour				✓		✓	✓	✓		✓
Cucumber	✓		✓	✓	✓	✓	✓	✓	✓	✓
Egg white			✓			✓			✓	
Egg yolk				✓		✓	✓	✓		✓
Flower waters	✓							✓	✓	✓

	Cleansing	Exfoliant	Toning	Moisturizing	+ Acid	Softening	Suncare	SKIN TYPE		
								Normal	Oily	Dry/Mature
Fuller's earth								☐	☐	☐
Glycerine				☐				☐	☐	☐
Grape			☐	☐	☐	☐		☐	☐	☐
Grapefruit		☐	☐		☐	☐		☐	☐	☐
Honey	☐		☐	☐		☐	☐	☐	☐	☐
Horseradish	☐		☐	☐	☐	☐		☐		☐
Jojoba oil	☐			☐		☐	☐	☐	☐	☐
Lanolin	☐			☐		☐		☐	☐	☐
Lemon	☐	☐	☐		☐			☐	☐	☐
Milk				☐		☐	☐	☐	☐	☐
Oatmeal	☐	☐	☐	☐		☐		☐	☐	☐
Olive oil	☐			☐		☐	☐	☐		☐
Peach				☐		☐	☐	☐	☐	☐
Petroleum jelly	☐					☐		☐	☐	☐
Pineapple	☐	☐	☐		☐	☐		☐	☐	☐
Rice flour	☐	☐				☐		☐	☐	☐
Sea salt		☐						☐	☐	
Strawberry			☐	☐	☐	☐	☐	☐	☐	☐
Vinegar, cider	☐	☐	☐	☐		☐		☐	☐	☐
Vinegar, wine	☐	☐	☐	☐		☐		☐	☐	☐
Wheat germ oil	☐			☐		☐	☐	☐		☐
Witch hazel	☐		☐			☐		☐	☐	☐
Yogurt	☐	☐	☐	☐	☐	☐		☐	☐	☐

FACE

cleanse

exfoliate

tone

moisturize

nourish

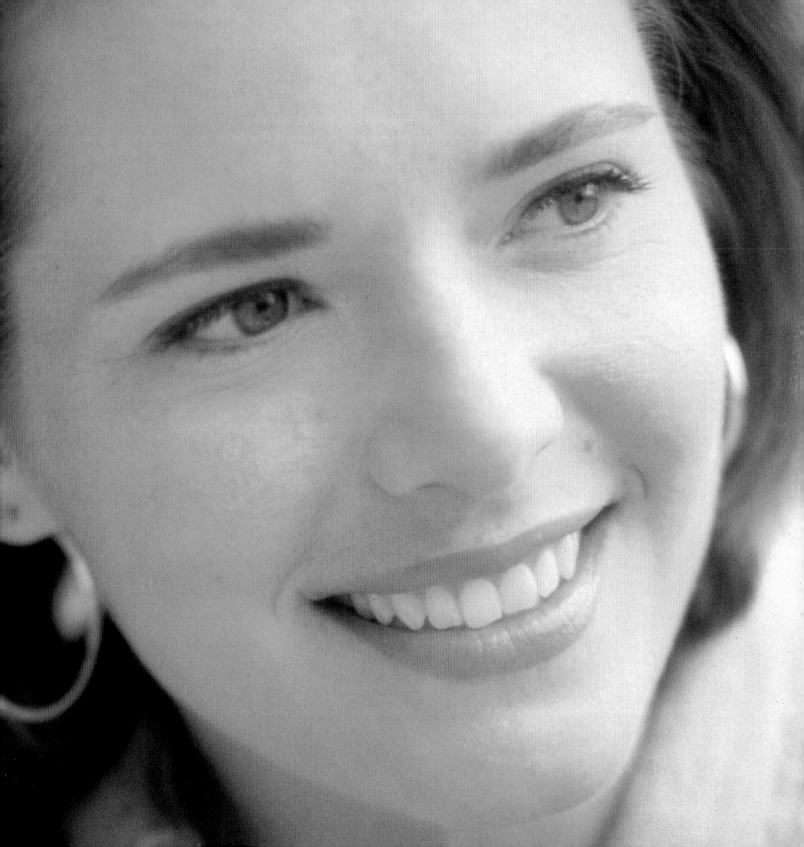

Your face is the part of you that you show to the world. It is also the part that is exposed to extremes of weather, to pollution, sunlight, and to the grime picked up through everyday living. You therefore have to make doubly sure that you take care of it.

The skin on a newborn baby is soft, smooth, and very elastic, and there is a high turnover of cells. As we age, the parts of us most exposed to the outside world

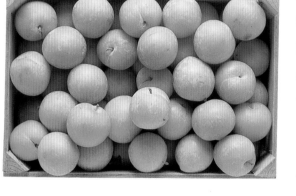

become coarser. This is largely due to the gradual slowing of the turnover of cells, which results in a buildup of dead cells on the surface of the skin. If we lavish plenty of time and attention on ourselves, some of the effects of aging can be kept at bay.

Hormone changes throughout life can affect our skin. At adolescence, the effect is nearly always to produce excess sebum. It always seems unfair that just as you are starting to be attracted to the opposite sex, you are very often suffering from oily skin, blackheads, or blemishes. During pregnancy skin seems to

glow with health, but afterwards hormone changes again may cause it to be extra oily or extra dry. It is probably at menopause that women notice the greatest change to their skin, as its natural elasticity begins to weaken.

Never give up on your skin and your appearance. No matter how old you are, there is always something that you can do to improve your looks, and to make yourself feel better.

FACIAL CARE

There are three basic, everyday steps to facial care. These are: cleansing, toning, and moisturizing. To this you can add: exfoliating, massage, and exercise. All of these are explained in the pages that follow.

All the instructions and recipes in this book are for skin treatments, not for makeup. Whether you wear a heavy makeup every day consisting of foundation and powder, is up to you. If you do, extra emphasis must be put on cleansing. Wearing no makeup is good for your skin as it lets it breathe and keeps the pores free. Try to set aside certain days in the week when your skin can be as nature intended.

And don't forget your neck! It is just below your face and still on show, so look after it. Include it in your cleansing, toning, and moisturizing routine, and try the special treatments on page 47.

Remember that when you start a program of facial care, the skin takes between three and four weeks to renew itself. You will probably have to wait that long to see clear results. Don't give up after a week or two because the treatment doesn't seem to be doing any good.

Assessing your skin type
Before you begin pampering your face, you must know what type of skin you have in order to choose the most suitable ingredients for your beauty preparations. Your basic skin type is usually inherited from your parents, but it is also affected by such things as diet, hormonal changes, and the atmosphere of your surroundings. Whether your skin is dry, normal, oily, or a combination type depends on how much sebum it produces.

Normal skin produces just enough sebum to keep the skin smooth and supple. Those people blessed with normal skin probably never even think about skin type, because their skin rarely poses a problem.

Oily skin produces more sebum than is needed and you may be able to feel a slight, greasy film on the surface. Where the sebaceous glands are overproductive, the acid mantle can become thick, clog the pores, and produce blackheads or cause acne. Oily skin is particularly noticeable over what is called the T-zone, the part of the face comprising the central strip and the forehead. Monthly hormonal changes often affect oily skin. But oily skin can be kept under control, especially if it is exfoliated regularly and you pay particular attention to your diet. It also has the advantage of not aging so quickly as dry or normal skin.

Dry skin is fine textured and thin and can become flaky and rough when exposed to extremes of temperature. It may be caused by insufficient sebum production or by dead cells on the surface failing to break up and so forming a scaly layer that in turn encourages a loss of moisture from the cells coming up. Rich nourishing creams and gentle exfoliation help.

Combination skin is a combination of normal and oily skin, the oily area being in the above mentioned T-zone. Each of the recipes is coded so that you can tell at a glance which ones will suit your skin: **N** normal, **D** dry, **O** oily, **P** problem, and **A** all types.

CLEANSING

By the end of a busy day, the skin on your face will have picked up a good deal of grime from the atmosphere, which mixes with dead skin cells, sebum, sweat, and any makeup you are wearing. If you did not cleanse your skin, every day more matter would build up, your pores would become clogged, and your skin would become dull and lifeless. Even traces of dirt left behind can cause problems, so proper daily cleansing should be built into your routine.

A quick wipe over with warm water will not be sufficient, although it is a good start and helps to get off the surface grime. Many people swear by soap and water, but soaps are often very alkaline and destroy the acid mantle of the skin. If you like soap, choose one that is gentle and specially made for the face.

Cleansing creams and oils are excellent for removing makeup and most of the daily grime and are mostly suitable for normal and dry skins. They do, however, leave a thin film of oil behind, so you should also use a facial scrub or steam from time to time. Oily skins need something lighter, and oil free.

Steaming

Along with everyday cleansing, your face needs a more thorough cleansing at regular intervals. Steaming is an excellent way of softening the skin and opening the pores to rid them of excess sebum. It can also soften blackheads, making them easier to remove. Even dry skin can benefit from steaming, particularly if it is followed by a massage using a nourishing oil.

The steam from plain water can moisturize and soften your skin. However, if the boiling water is poured over dried or chopped herbs, the properties of the herbs will be released.

It is best not to steam too frequently since, after all, it does subject your delicate facial skin to an unusual heat. Once a week is fine for normal or oily skin; every two weeks if you have dry skin. Do not steam your face if you have broken veins. See page 33 for instructions on how best to steam and deep clean your skin.

HERBS FOR STEAMING

Choose one of the following herbs, or refer to the chart on page 19.

All skin types
Chamomile, comfrey, elderflower, linden flower, nettle

Normal or dry skin
Lady's mantle, marshmallow

Normal or oily skin
Fennel, lemon balm, rosemary

Oily skin
Sage, mint, yarrow

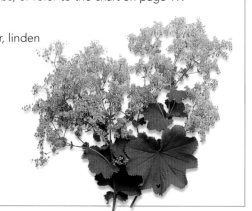

Gently massage one of these simple skin cleansers into the skin, then rinse off with lukewarm water or an herbal infusion chosen to suit your skin type.

• Buttermilk; cornmeal, ground almonds, or fine oatmeal made into a paste with mineral water; plain yogurt on its own or mixed with a little herbal infusion (all skin types); for oily skin, mix plain yogurt with a little lemon juice; use dried milk powder, moistened with water on normal or oily skin, and whole milk on normal or dry skin.

RECIPE

HERBAL WITCH HAZEL CLEANSER Ⓐ

A light, liquid cleansing lotion that is excellent for wiping away daily grime. Soak a cotton ball in the lotion and wipe it gently over your face. Choose a herb to suit your skin type.

1 tsp dried or 1 tbsp fresh chopped chosen herb

⅓ cup/90 ml boiling water

4 tbsp/60 ml witch hazel

2 tbsp/30 ml glycerine

1 Place the herb in a bowl and pour on the boiling water. Cover and leave to cool. Strain.
2 Pour 2 tbsp/30 ml of the infusion into a sterilized bottle or jar. Add the witch hazel and glycerine. Cover tightly and shake well.
3 Store in a refrigerator and use within one week. Shake before use.

RECIPE

BUTTERMILK AND HONEY CLEANSER Ⓝ Ⓓ

Buttermilk is very soothing for the face. The herbs used here are for normal to dry skin. For an oily skin, use yarrow, sage or horsetail, or a mixture of two of them.

⅔ cup/150 ml buttermilk

1 tbsp dried or 1 tsp fresh elderflowers

1 tsp dried or 1 tbsp fresh linden flowers

1 tsp honey

1 Place the buttermilk and herbs in a saucepan. Cover and leave for two hours.
2 Set the pan on a low heat and bring the mixture gently to a boil.
3 Remove from the heat, stir in the honey and leave to cool.
4 Strain off the liquid and pour it into a sterilized bottle. Seal and store in a refrigerator. Use within five days.

LINDEN OR LIME TREE (*Tilea vulgaris*)

Linden or lime trees grow wild, and in parks and gardens, throughout the northern temperate zones of the world. Infusions and decoctions of linden flowers are very emollient and can be used for all skin types.

Linden trees are common in Britain and Europe. More common in the eastern United States is basswood (*Tilea americana*), which can be used in the same ways as linden.

Other traditional names for the linden are lime tree, line, linn flowers, pry, and whitewood.

The sweetly scented yellow-green flowers of the linden are usually ready for picking and drying in midsummer. You can sometimes buy dried linden flowers, but if they are unavailable, buy linden flower tea bags. (Make sure that no other ingredients have been added to the tea bags.)

MILK AND CUCUMBER CLEANSER ⓝ ⓞ

This cleanser is for normal to oily skin. It is cooling and refreshing and leaves your skin feeling very smooth.

2 in/5 cm piece cucumber

⅓ cup/90 ml milk

4 drops tincture of benzoin

1 Peel and chop the cucumber.
2 Place the cucumber in a blender or food processor. Add the milk and work until smooth.
3 Pour the mixture into a saucepan and set on a medium heat. Bring to simmering point and hold there for two minutes.
4 Remove from the heat and allow to cool. Strain.
5 Pour the liquid into a sterilized bottle and add the tincture of benzoin.
6 Store in a refrigerator and use within one week.

YOGURT CLEANSER ⓐ

Yogurt acts as a skin food as well as a cleanser, and leaves your skin feeling smooth. Choose a herb to suit your skin type.

1 tsp dried or 1 tbsp fresh chopped chosen herb

⅓ cup/90 ml boiling water

5 tbsp/75 ml plain yogurt

1 tsp/5 ml lemon juice (for oily skin)

1 tsp/5 ml wheat germ oil (for dry to normal skin)

1 Place the herb in a bowl and pour on the boiling water. Cover and leave to cool. Strain.
2 Place the yogurt in a bowl and gradually beat in the infusion. Add the lemon juice or wheat germ oil.
3 Store in a sterilized jar in a refrigerator and use within one week. Shake before using, especially if using oil.

ALMOND MILK CLEANSER ⓐ

Almond milk is a time-honored beauty treatment. Crushing the almonds by hand is said to draw out more "milk," but you can use a blender or food processor instead. The cleanser is suitable for all skin types.

6 tbsp whole almonds

cold water

2 tsp/10 ml honey

¾ cup/200 ml mineral water

4 tbsp/60 ml rosewater

1 Place the almonds in a saucepan and cover them with cold water. Bring to a boil. Allow to cool. Strain, then squeeze the almonds from their skins when still moist.
2 Chop the almonds finely by hand or in a blender or food processor.
3 Crush the almonds by hand using a large, heavy mortar and pestle.
4 Transfer the almonds to a bowl and beat in the honey. Add the mineral water, a few tablespoons at a time. Cover and leave to stand for eight hours.
5 Strain off the liquid through muslin, squeezing well to extract as much as possible.
6 Add the rosewater.
7 Store in a sterilized bottle or jar in a refrigerator. Use within three weeks.

ALMONDS

In medieval times, almond milk, made by soaking, simmering, and straining pulverized almonds, was used for both culinary and beauty purposes when ordinary milk was scarce. This was often the case during the winter months or during Lent, when the use of cow's milk was forbidden.

SOAPWORT CLEANSER Ⓐ

Keep in the bathroom and use directly from the bottle, as a gentle facewash. It will lather like soap but will leave your skin feeling soft. After use, rinse with warm water and pat dry.

1 tbsp soapwort root

2 tbsp dried or 6 tbsp fresh chopped chosen herb

3 pints/1.5 liters water, preferably mineral water

1 Place the soapwort root and herb in a saucepan with the water and cover. Bring gently to a boil and simmer for five minutes.
2 Take the pan from the heat and leave the decoction to cool.
3 Strain, pressing down well, and bottle the liquid. Use within one month.

SOAPWORT (*Saponaria officinalis*) AND SOAPBARK (*Quillaja saponaria*)

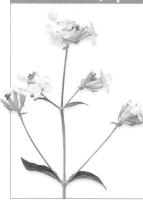

Soapwort is the mildest form of cleanser for any skin type. When the dried root is simmered in water, it produces a decoction that will lather slightly when used as a wash. It can safely be used as a substitute for face and body soap, or as a wash for the hair.

Soapbark can be used in the same ways as soapwort. The bark of the tree produces a foamy liquid when boiled. It was once used to make foamy soft drinks, but is now just used externally, and as a fabric cleaner. Soapbark grows in South America, most particularly in Chile, and is a member of the wing-seeded section of the rose family. It is an evergreen tree with thick, toothed, oval, shiny green leaves and white flowers. It can grow up to 60 ft (18 m) high, and is also known as Panama Bark Tree and Cullay.

COCOA BUTTER CLEANSER Ⓓ

This is an excellent lotion for dry skin. It enriches and moisturizes the area around the eyes as it cleanses. Mineral water may be used instead of the elderflower infusion.

1 tbsp elderflowers

⅔ cup/150 ml boiling water

1 tbsp/15 ml cocoa butter

1 tbsp/15 ml lanolin

½ cup/125 ml almond or olive oil

1 Place the elderflowers in a pitcher and pour on the boiling water. Cover and leave to cool. Strain.
2 Place the cocoa butter, lanolin and oil in the top part of a double boiler or into a bowl set in a saucepan of water. Melt together over a low heat.
3 Remove the mixture from the heat and add 3 tbsp/45 ml of the elderflower infusion.
4 Whisk the mixture until it is well blended and cool.
5 Transfer the lotion to a sterilized pot or jar. Cover when completely cold. Use within three months.

LIGHT BEESWAX CLEANSER Ⓐ

This is a light textured cleansing cream, suitable for all skin types. For normal and dry skin use rosewater or an infusion of elderflowers or marigolds; for oily skin, use chamomile or yarrow.

1 tbsp/15 ml beeswax

1 tbsp/15 ml white petroleum jelly

4 tbsp/60 ml almond oil

2 tbsp/30 ml rosewater or herbal infusion

2-3 drops essential oil such as rose or lavender (only if using infusion)

1 Place the beeswax, petroleum jelly, and almond oil in the top of a double boiler or into a bowl set in a saucepan of water. Melt them gently together on a low heat.
2 Warm the rosewater or infusion.
3 Remove entirely from the heat and beat the rosewater or infusion into the beeswax mixture. Leave to cool.
4 Transfer the cream to a sterilized pot or jar. Cover when completely cold. Use within three months.

ALMOND AND IRISH MOSS CLEANSER ◉

In texture this is rather like soft modeling clay, and spreads easily over the face. Spread it on with your fingers and remove with soft tissues or cotton balls.

⅔ cup/150 ml hot water

½ tsp borax

2 tsp Irish moss

1 tbsp/15 ml almond oil

2 tbsp ground almonds

1 In a bowl, dissolve the borax in the hot water.
2 Add the Irish moss and leave to soak for four hours, or until it becomes soft and jellylike.
3 Mix together the almonds and oil.
4 Stir them vigorously into the Irish moss.
5 Store in a sterilized pot or jar in a refrigerator. Use within two weeks.

IRISH MOSS (*Chondrus crispus*)

Irish moss, or carragheen, is a seaweed that grows in purple-brown fan shapes on rocks or in rock pools below the tide line. It is harvested in the spring and dried. When mixed with water and soaked or simmered, it forms a jellylike mucilage that can be used as a base for desserts or for medicinal and beauty purposes.

HERBAL COLD CREAM Ⓐ

The ancient recipe for cold cream has remained the same for nearly 2,000 years. It is suitable for all skin types, particularly if an herbal infusion to match your skin is used as the liquid.

1 tbsp dried chosen herb to suit skin

⅔ cup/150 ml boiling water

¼ tsp borax

1 tbsp/15 ml beeswax

⅓ cup/90 ml almond oil

1 drop rose or other suitable essential oil

1 Place the herb in a pitcher and pour in the boiling water. Cover and leave to cool slightly. Strain.
2 Dissolve the borax in 4 tbsp/60 ml of the warm infusion.
3 Place the wax and oil in the top of a double boiler or in a bowl set in a saucepan of water. Set on a low heat and melt the wax and oil.
4 Beat in the infusion, then add the rose or other essential oil.
5 Remove entirely from the heat and beat vigorously with a wooden spoon or an electric beater, until the mixture is cool and creamy in texture.
6 Transfer the cream to a sterilized pot or jar. Cover when completely cold. Use within three months.

COLD CREAM

Cold cream was invented by Galen, personal physician to the Emperor Marcus Aurelius around AD 170. In the sixteenth century it was prepared with oil of cole-seed and called "cole cream," which later became "cold cream." It has been used as a moisturizer and a cleanser and, in the sixteenth century, it was spread on cloth and used as a night-time face mask.

APRICOT AND AVOCADO CLEANSER Ⓝ Ⓓ

This light-textured, cream should be used at night as a combined cleanser and enriching oil. Leave the residue to nourish your skin as you sleep.

4 tbsp/60 ml apricot oil

4 tbsp/60 ml avocado oil

2 tbsp/30 ml chosen herbal infusion or mineral water

1 Beat all the ingredients together with an electric beater. The mixture should be light, white, and creamy in texture.
2 Transfer to a sterilized bottle or jar and cover. Shake well before use. Use within two months.

RICH MARIGOLD CLEANSER Ⓝ Ⓓ

This makes a very soft cream that is suitable for normal or dry, sensitive skins.

4 fresh or dried marigold heads

1 tbsp/15 ml cocoa butter

1 tbsp/15 ml lanolin

½ cup/125 ml almond, avocado, apricot, or olive oil

1 Place all the ingredients in the top part of a double boiler or into a bowl set in a pan of water. Set them on a low heat and let the cocoa butter, lanolin, and oil melt together.
2 Leave on a low heat for a further five minutes.
3 Strain the mixture through a sieve into another bowl and beat until it cools.
4 Transfer the cream to a sterilized pot or jar. Cover when completely cold. Use within three months.

MARIGOLD (*Calendula officinalis*)

The marigold, or calendula, has been valued for its soothing and healing properties for centuries. It came originally from southern Europe, but was soon taken north to become well known to the Anglo-Saxons. The Spaniards took the marigold to Mexico where it was believed to have sprung from the blood of natives killed by the invaders. Early settlers took it to North America; it was later used to heal wounds by both sides in the American Civil War.

Marigolds have always been popular because they are easy to grow and exceptionally useful. They heal wounds, soothe chilblains (see page 114) and insect bites, and can be made into a compress for bruises and sprains.

EXFOLIATING

Exfoliation is the process by which unwanted dead cells are removed from the surface of the skin to encourage new growth and a healthy glow. The value of exfoliants for all skin types has been recognized only in the last few years.

Five hundred million dead cells rub off us daily, and it has been found that gently assisting their departure helps to speed up the production of new cells and improve blood circulation in the skin. So if your skin looks dull and uneven, remove the top layer with a mild exfoliant to make it smooth, shiny, and glowing.

Unless you have a medical skin complaint, you will benefit from exfoliation. A dry skin, for example, is often only dry because the outer layer of dead cells cling persistently together and cannot break down. If you give it a regular helping hand, the skin's surface will no longer be dry and may become normal.

It is never too late to begin exfoliating your skin. If you get into the habit early, then your skin will benefit for the rest of your life. As you get older, the rate of cell replacement in your skin slows down naturally, but regular exfoliation will give it a boost and may keep you looking younger for a little longer.

If you have never tried an exfoliant on your skin before, it is best to start with the milder ingredients such as oatmeal, buttermilk, and ground almonds. If your skin benefits from the treatment and there are no ill effects, try adding small amounts of fruit, such as pineapple or lemon, to find the ingredients that suit you best.

Face masks

Homemade face masks have many uses, both direct and indirect. They have a beneficial effect on the skin of the face and this can be cleansing, moisturizing, healing, tautening or exfoliating. Their secondary effect is brought about by the fact that you generally have to lie down while they take effect. If you walk about, they may slither downwards. You can't even talk when wearing those that harden on the skin. So relax, lie down, and make this a part of the treatment, too.

Face masks have to be of a spreadable consistency that will stay on the face. Some, as mentioned above, are designed to dry and harden, others change very little. They are all made from a base substance into which other ingredients are mixed.

Base substances include cereals, such as oatmeal, cornmeal, rice flour, barley and bran, and natural powders such as fuller's earth or

EXFOLIATION

What you will need:

Bowl large enough to hold 2½ cups/575 ml boiling water

1 tbsp dried or 3 tbsp fresh chopped herbs

Face mask or scrub chosen from the recipes found on pages 35-36

2-3 medium sized towels

Face cloth

Toner and moisturizer chosen to suit skin type

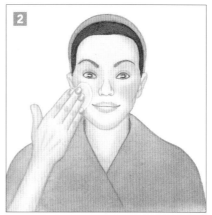

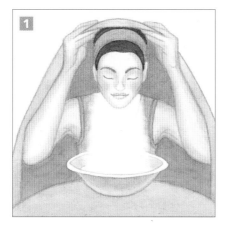

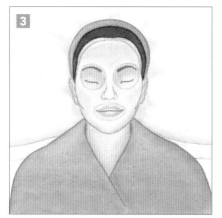

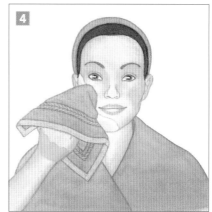

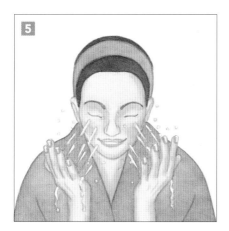

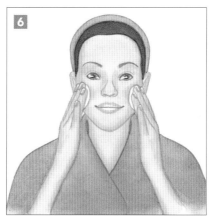

1 Place the herb in the bowl and pour on the boiling water. Cover your head and the bowl with the towel, and close your eyes. Keep your face 1 ft/30 cm above the water for 10-15 minutes.

2 Prepare your chosen scrub or mask, then tie back your hair and wrap a towel around your shoulders. Using the tips of your fingers, spread the mixture in an even layer over your face and neck, avoiding the sensitive part around your eyes. If you have chosen a scrub, massage it into your skin then go to step 4.

3 If using a face mask, lie down and relax for fifteen minutes. (First cover a pillow with another towel.) Breathe deeply and enjoy this special time.

4 Wipe away the scrub. When the mask treatment is finished, come back to the world slowly. Gently wipe away the mask with a face cloth.

5 Rinse off the remaining mask or scrub with lukewarm water and pat your face dry.

6 Apply a toner and apply a suitable moisturizer while your skin is still slightly damp.

kaolin. Ground almonds could also be included in this section. These are dry and powdery and have to be moistened. Moisteners include small amounts of natural oils, dairy products such as buttermilk, milk, yogurt or cream, egg (either whole or separated), fruit or vegetable purées or herbal infusions.

Exfoliants can be used either as a facial scrub or as a mask. A scrub is useful when time is short, a mask takes longer and is more relaxing. For a deep-cleansing effect, steam your face first.

TONING

After cleansing, steaming, or exfoliating, the skin must be toned to cool it down and help it to contract. Toners reduce any grease left behind by oil-based cleansers; they help to dry oily skin and leave it feeling cool and fresh.

MOISTURIZING

Water is essential in maintaining a healthy skin. Drinking eight glasses of water a day will help, but you can also add moisture from the outside. A good moisturizing treatment should both moisturize and nourish. It should add water to the skin's surface and should also help to reinforce the thin oily layer on the skin called the hydrolipidic film, which helps to keep the moisture from disappearing into the surrounding atmosphere.

Moisturizing comes after cleansing and toning. It is a good idea to massage the moisturizer into your skin before the toner is completely dry, thus keeping in even more moisture. Spread the mixture onto your face with your fingertips, using some of the facial

(Continued on page 38.)

HERBS FOR TONING

Normal skin

Chamomile, dandelion, elderflower, fennel, lemon balm, marigold, parsley, rosemary

Oily skin

Choose from herbs listed for normal skin, or any of the following: Horsetail, lady's mantle, peppermint, sage, yarrow

Dry skin

Elderflower, linden flowers, marigold, marshmallow (Mix the infusion half and half with rosewater.)

OATMEAL

Oatmeal has been used for centuries as a natural cleanser and softener. When moistened and rubbed into the skin it dislodges surface cells and embedded dirt as well as cleansing the pores. It also contains proteins that nourish and soften the skin at the same time. Oatmeal is a very mild skin treatment that can be used on all skin types, including sensitive skins and on skins that have acne.

GROUND ALMOND AND HONEY FACIAL SCRUB Ⓐ

This is a mild exfoliant and a good one to start with. The rose oil is not essential, but it makes a luxurious preparation if added. Do not use a synthetic rose oil.

2 tbsp ground almonds

2 tsp/10 ml honey

4 tbsp/60 ml buttermilk or plain yogurt

2 drops rose oil

1 Place the ground almonds and honey in a bowl.
2 Mix in the buttermilk to make a thick paste.
3 Beat in the rose oil.
4 Gently massage the mixture into your face and neck for about two minutes, avoiding the area directly around the eyes.
5 Rinse off the mixture with tepid water. Pat dry, tone, and moisturize.

HERBAL FACIAL SCRUB Ⓐ

This is very mild and gentle, and so another good scrub to begin with.

herbal infusion made with chamomile, elderflowers, or fennel

2 tbsp fine oatmeal

1 Mix 3 tbsp/45 ml of the infusion with the oatmeal to make a paste. Leave the oatmeal to soften for five minutes.
2 Gently massage the mixture into your face for five minutes.
3 Rinse off the mixture with tepid water. Pat dry, tone, and moisturize.

OATMEAL AND YOGURT FACIAL SCRUB Ⓓ Ⓟ

The almond oil makes this an ideal scrub for dry skin, leaving it feeling soft and smooth. Without the almond oil, the exfoliant is suitable for skin that suffers from acne.

2 tbsp fine oatmeal

2 tbsp/30 ml plain yogurt

1 tbsp/15 ml almond oil

1 Place the oatmeal in a bowl and gradually mix in the yogurt and almond oil. Leave the oatmeal to soften for five minutes.
2 Gently massage the mixture into your face and neck for about five minutes, avoiding the area directly around the eyes.
3 Rinse off with tepid water, pat dry, tone, and moisturize.

CORNMEAL FACIAL SCRUB Ⓞ

Cornmeal exfoliators are good for oily skins, and the lemon juice adds to the acid mantle.

2 tbsp cornmeal

1 tsp/5 ml lemon juice

2 tbsp/30 ml plain yogurt or buttermilk

1 Place the cornmeal in a bowl.
2 Mix in the lemon juice and buttermilk to make a paste. Leave the cornmeal to soften for five minutes.
3 Gently massage the paste into your face for about five minutes, avoiding the area around the eyes.
4 Rinse off the mixture with tepid water. Pat dry, tone, and moisturize.

GRAPEFRUIT AND PARSLEY FACE MASK Ⓞ

This leaves your skin feeling new and refreshed. Parsley is particularly good for oily skin.

3 tbsp fine oatmeal

2 tbsp chopped parsley

juice of ½ large grapefruit

1 Place the oatmeal and parsley in a bowl.
2 Mix in enough grapefruit juice to make a spreadable paste. Let soften for five minutes.
3 Spread the mixture evenly over your face.
4 Lie down and relax for 15 minutes.
5 Rinse off the mixture with tepid water. Pat dry, tone, and moisturize.

PINEAPPLE AND CORNMEAL FACE MASK ◎

Pineapple leaves your skin feeling fresh and slightly taut. Like the previous cornmeal recipe, this is good for oily skins.

1 slice pineapple, ½ inch/1.3 cm thick

2 tbsp/30 ml plain yogurt

4 tbsp cornmeal

1 Purée the pineapple slice in a food processor or blender.
2 Put the purée into a bowl and mix in the yogurt and enough cornmeal to make a thick paste. Leave it for five minutes for the cornmeal to soften.
3 Spread the paste over your face, avoiding the area immediately around the eyes.
4 Lie down and relax for 15 minutes.
5 Rinse off the mixture with tepid water, pat dry, tone, and moisturize.

PINEAPPLE

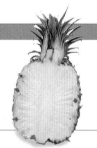

Pineapple is a natural exfoliant. It contains a protein-digesting enzyme called bromelin that gently breaks down the dead skin cells so they can be easily removed, leaving your skin feeling soft and smooth. Pineapple also restores the skin's natural acid mantle. Pineapple slices can be puréed and made into face masks or scrubs. You can also lay thin slices on your face while you lie down and relax.

HERBAL MILK TONER ⓓ ⓟ

Skin toners made with milk are soothing and nourishing for dry, sunburned, or sensitive skins. Choose whole milk for dry or normal skin, skim milk for oily skins.

2 tsp dried or 1 tbsp fresh chopped herb chosen to suit skin type

⅔ cup/150 ml milk

1 Place the herb in a bowl or pitcher.
2 Boil the milk and pour it over the herb. Cover and leave until cold.
3 Strain through muslin or cheesecloth.
4 Store in a sterilized bottle or jar in a refrigerator. Use within five days.

HERB AND WITCH HAZEL TONER ⓐ

This is a light, refreshing toner for all skin types that is very easy to make.

1 tsp dried or 1 tbsp fresh chopped herb chosen to suit skin type

⅓ cup/90 ml boiling water

2 tbsp/30 ml witch hazel

pinch boric acid

1 Place the herb in a bowl or pitcher and pour on the boiling water. Cover and leave to cool. Strain.
2 Mix the boric acid into the witch hazel.
3 Add the witch hazel to the herbal infusion.
4 Store in a sterilized bottle or jar in a refrigerator and use within one month. Shake well before use.

EGG WHITE AND LEMON TONER ◎

This is a toner for oily skin.

1 tbsp dried or 2 tbsp fresh chopped yarrow, horsetail, or sage

⅔ cup/150 ml boiling water

1 egg white

juice ½ lemon, strained

1 Place the herb in a pitcher or bowl and pour on the boiling water. Cover and leave to cool. Strain.
2 Whisk the egg white and lemon juice together.
3 Mix in the herbal infusion.
4 Store in a sterilized bottle or jar in a refrigerator. Use within one week.

• The simplest toner is cold water, rosewater, or orange-flower water, or a cold herbal infusion. Other things to wipe on your face include a slice of cucumber or the inside of a cucumber peel (all skin types); a cut strawberry (normal or oily skin). You may need to wash off any strawberry stains left on your skin, but the other toners can be left to dry.

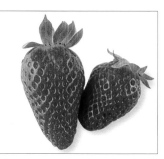

RECIPE

CITRUS TONER Ⓝ Ⓞ

This is a deliciously scented toner that freshens and clears normal to oily skin.

peel from 2 lemons, 2 oranges, and 1 grapefruit

1¼ cups/275 ml mineral water

2 tbsp/30 ml vodka (optional, but it doubles the shelf-life)

1 Place the citrus peels in a pitcher or bowl and pour on the mineral water. Cover and leave for 12 hours.
2 Strain the liquid through a coffee filter and into a sterilized bottle or jar. Add the vodka. Store in a refrigerator and use within two weeks (four weeks if vodka is added).

RECIPE

ALMOND TONER Ⓞ

This is an astringent toner, good for oily skins.

⅔ cup/150 ml rosewater

½ tsp borax

1 tsp/5 ml tincture of benzoin

1 tsp ground almonds

3 tbsp/45 ml mineral water or distilled water

1 Place the rosewater in a sterilized bottle or jar.
2 Dissolve the borax in the tincture of benzoin and add to the rosewater.
3 Mix the almonds with the water and add to the rosewater. Shake well.
4 Store in a refrigerator and use within one month. Shake before using.

RECIPE

CUCUMBER AND ELDERFLOWER TONER Ⓐ

This cooling and refreshing toner can be used for all skin types. The vodka prevents the cucumber from going moldy.

1 cucumber

3 tbsp dried elderflowers or 3 fresh heads

½ cup/125 ml boiling water

⅓ cup/90 ml vodka

1 Slice the cucumber. Place the slices into a saucepan with no water and set them on a low heat. Simmer until soft. Allow to cool then strain off the liquid through muslin, squeezing to extract as much liquid as possible.
2 Place the elderflowers in a pitcher or bowl and pour on the boiling water. Cover and leave to cool. Strain off the infusion.
3 Add the vodka and the infusion to the cucumber juice. Store in a refrigerator and use within two weeks.

CUCUMBER

The cucumber contains a large proportion of water, and so is naturally moisturizing. It also has the same acid-alkaline balance as the skin itself, making it one of the gentlest and most balanced of beauty treatments. Cucumber is used to moisturize and tone, and to ease sunburn and the effects of the weather.

massage techniques shown on page 50. Remember to moisturize your neck as well.

If you have normal skin, use a light moisturizer in the daytime and a richer one for overnight.

If you live and work in air-conditioned areas, or if you spend a lot of your time outdoors, you are more likely to have dry skin. Dry skins often do not produce enough sebum to maintain the acid mantle and so twice a day nourishing and moisturizing are particularly important. Use rich, oil-based moisturizers, and consider patting extra wheat germ or another natural vegetable oil into the skin at night after using the moisturizer.

Oily skin may not need moisturizing twice a day or even every day. As a replacement use a toner that moisturizes but which is not too astringent, and let it dry naturally. Examples are those made from one of the emollient herbs, such as linden flower or elderflower, or from rosewater and witch hazel. Try "Herb and witch hazel," "Cucumber and elderflower," or "Almond" from the toner recipes on pages 36-37. When you need to moisturize, use a light moisturizing lotion. If you have been out in the sun and wind all day and your skin feels dry, do use a rich moisturizer or massage in some jojoba or avocado oil.

Quick Fixes

If the skin on your face feels slack, try a face mask that will both tone and tauten.

• For normal or dry skin, apply a lightly beaten egg white and leave it to dry on your face. Adding 1 tbsp skim milk powder will soften your skin; 1 tsp/5 ml honey will moisturize.

• For very oily skin, beat the egg white with either 1 tbsp/15 ml lemon juice or cider vinegar.

• Add 2 tbsp fresh chopped herbs to the beaten white, for example parsley for normal skin and mint for oily skin.

RECIPE

CUCUMBER AND COCONUT MOISTURIZER Ⓝ Ⓓ

This soft, pale-green cream is suitable for dry or normal skins. You can feel the moisture of the cucumber as you spread it over your face.

3 in/7.5 cm piece cucumber

pinch borax

1 tsp/5 ml lanolin

1 tsp/5 ml cocoa butter

1 tbsp/15 ml beeswax

2 tbsp/30 ml coconut oil

1 Finely chop the cucumber and press it in a sieve to extract the juice. There should be about 2 tbsp/30 ml.
2 Warm the juice and dissolve the borax in it.
3 Place the lanolin, cocoa butter, beeswax, and coconut oil in the top of a double boiler or in a bowl set in a saucepan of water. Melt on a low heat.
4 Remove entirely from the heat and beat in the cucumber juice until the mixture is cool.
5 Transfer the cream to a sterilized pot or jar. Cover when completely cold. Use within six weeks.

VITAMIN-ENRICHED MOISTURIZER Ⓝ Ⓓ

Use this rich, creamy textured, yellow moisture cream for dry or normal skin types under makeup or overnight. Rosewater can be substituted for the herbal decoction.

1 tsp dried or 1 tbsp fresh chopped herb chosen to suit skin type

²⁄₃ cup/150 ml water

2 tbsp/30 ml lanolin

2 tbsp/30 ml beeswax

2 tbsp/30 ml wheat germ oil

¹⁄₃ cup/90 ml almond, avocado or olive oil

one 250 iu capsule vitamin E

one 250 iu capsule vitamin A

3 drops essential oil such as rose, lavender, or geranium (optional)

1 Place the herb and water in a saucepan and bring to a boil. Cover and simmer for five minutes. Leave to cool, then strain off the decoction.
2 Place the lanolin and beeswax in the top of a double boiler or in a bowl set in a saucepan of water. Melt gently on a low heat.
3 Gradually beat in the oils.
4 Remove entirely from the heat and beat in 2 tbsp/30 ml of the herbal decoction or rosewater.
5 Pierce the vitamin capsules and squeeze the contents into the cream. Beat well, adding the essential oil, if using.
6 Cool, stirring frequently.
7 Transfer the cream to a sterilized pot or jar. Cover when completely cold. Use within two months.

COCOA BUTTER MOISTURIZER Ⓓ

Rosewater can be substituted for the herbal decoction in this rich, fairly stiff, cream.

1 tsp dried or 1 tbsp fresh chopped herb chosen to suit skin type

²⁄₃ cup/150 ml water

3 tbsp/45 ml cocoa butter

1 tbsp/15 ml beeswax

½ cup/125 ml almond, avocado, olive, or safflower oil

3 drops essential oil such as rose, lavender, or geranium (optional)

1 Place the herb and water in a saucepan and bring to a boil. Cover and simmer for five minutes. Leave to cool, then strain off the decoction.
2 Place the cocoa butter and beeswax in the top of a double boiler or in a bowl set in a saucepan of water. Melt gently on a low heat.
3 Gradually beat in the oil.
4 Remove entirely from the heat and beat in 2 tbsp/30 ml of the herbal decoction or rosewater. Add the essential oil, if using.
5 Cool, stirring frequently.
6 Transfer the cream to a sterilized pot or jar. Cover when completely cold. Use within two months.

GERANIUM OIL

Geranium oil is revitalizing and relaxing. It is produced, mainly in countries around the Mediterranean, by a steam distillation of the leaves and flowers of a species of pelargonium.

The scent of geranium oil combines an herbal freshness with an underlying sweetness, and it is often used to scent soaps, creams and perfumes.

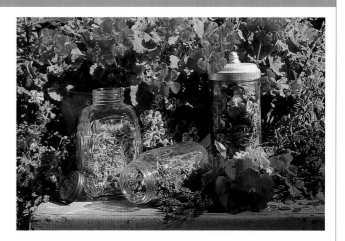

HONEY AND OLIVE OIL MOISTURIZER ⓝ ⓓ

This light-colored cream suits dry or normal skin. Rosewater can be substituted for the herbal infusion

1 tsp dried or 1 tbsp fresh chopped herb chosen to suit skin type

⅔ cup/150 ml water

1 tbsp/15 ml beeswax

2 tbsp/30 ml lanolin

⅓ cup/90 ml olive oil

2 tsp/10 ml honey

2 drops essential oil such as rose, lavender, or geranium (optional)

1 Place the herb and water in a saucepan and bring to a boil. Cover and simmer for five minutes. Leave to cool, then strain off the decoction.
2 Place the beeswax and lanolin in the top of a double boiler or in a bowl set in a saucepan of water. Melt gently on a low heat.
3 Gradually beat in the oil.
4 Remove entirely from the heat and beat in the honey and 2 tbsp/30 ml of the herbal decoction or rosewater. Add the essential oil, if using.
5 Cool, stirring frequently.
6 Transfer the cream to a sterilized pot or jar. Cover when completely cold. Use within two months.

ELDERFLOWER SKIN NOURISHER ⓓ

In texture this is like a thick lotion rather than a cream, and spreads very easily over the skin.

3 tbsp dried or 3 heads fresh elderflowers

½ cup/125 ml almond, olive, or safflower oil

2 tbsp/30 ml lanolin

1 Place all the ingredients in the top of a double boiler or in a bowl set in a saucepan of water. Let the lanolin and oil melt together, then keep on a very low heat for 30 minutes.
2 Strain the cream into a small, sterilized pot or jar. Cover when completely cold.

ELDERFLOWER (*Sambucus nigra*)

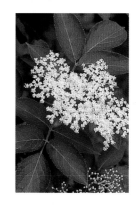

The elder tree grows in woods, on abandoned land, and often near walls of old or derelict cottages throughout Europe. There are two related species in North America. The American or sweet elder (*Sambucus canadensis*), which is sometimes called elderblow, grows in the midwestern and eastern United States, the Plains states and Texas. The blue berried elder (*Sambucus glauca*) grows mainly in the extreme western states and is cultivated as an ornamental tree along the Pacific coast.

The creamy-white flower heads of all these trees can be used for cosmetic purposes. Infusions or decoctions of elderflower have a soothing and emollient effect on the skin, and are suitable for all skin types.

CUCUMBER MOISTURIZER ⓐ

This is good for all skin types. It is a nice green color and feels very soothing and refreshing when patted onto the skin.

4 in/10 cm piece cucumber

⅓ cup/90 ml rosewater

3 tbsp/45 ml glycerine

1 Finely chop or blend the cucumber, then press it in a sieve to extract the juice.
2 Place the juice, rosewater, and glycerine into a sterilized bottle, cover and shake together.
3 Store in a refrigerator and use within one week. Shake well before using.

RECIPE

MARIGOLD MOISTURIZER Ⓝ Ⓓ

Use this rich lotion for normal to dry skins and for skins that have been exposed to the sun or wind. The oils will separate from the liquid, but a quick, vigorous shake before use will amalgamate the lotion for a short time.

2 tbsp dried marigolds or 6 fresh marigold heads

⅔ cup/150 ml water

1 tsp/5 ml cocoa butter

1 tsp/5 ml lanolin

4 tbsp/60 ml sesame or olive oil

1 Place the marigold in a saucepan with the water and bring to a boil. Cover and simmer for ten minutes. Strain off the decoction.
2 Place the cocoa butter, lanolin, and oil in the top of a double boiler or in a bowl set in a saucepan of water. Melt them together.
3 Remove entirely from the heat then gradually beat in the marigold infusion. Leave until cold.
4 Transfer the lotion to a sterilized bottle and shake well. Use within six weeks. Shake before use.

RECIPE

ROSEWATER MOISTURIZER Ⓐ

This is rich and refreshing at the same time. Like the marigold lotion, the oils will separate, so the lotion will always need a quick shake before use.

1 tsp/5 ml cocoa butter

1 tsp/5 ml lanolin

4 tbsp/60 ml sesame or olive oil

⅓ cup/90 ml rosewater

2 tbsp/30 ml witch hazel

1 Place the cocoa butter, lanolin, and oil in the top of a double boiler or in a bowl set in a saucepan of water. Melt them together.
2 Gradually beat in the rosewater.
3 Remove entirely from the heat and stir in the witch hazel. Leave until cold.
4 Transfer the lotion to a sterilized bottle and shake well. Use within six weeks. Shake before use.

RECIPE

OILY SKIN MOISTURIZER Ⓞ

Oily skin needs a moisturizer that will not add to its oiliness. Yarrow, sage, and tincture of benzoin are efficient astringents, and the glycerine provides all the lubrication required.

1 tsp dried or 1 tbsp fresh chopped yarrow or sage

⅔ cup/150 ml water

⅓ cup/90 ml rosewater

2 tbsp/30 ml glycerine

1 tbsp/15 ml witch hazel

½ tsp/5 ml tincture of benzoin

1 Place the herb in a saucepan with the water and bring to a boil. Cover and simmer for ten minutes. Cool and strain.
2 Transfer the herbal decoction to a sterilized bottle or jar and add the remaining ingredients. Cover and shake well. Use within two months. Shake well before use.

YARROW (Achillea millefolium)

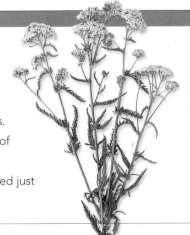

Yarrow grows wild in Europe, and throughout North America. In Australia, it is mainly found in cultivation, but it frequently escapes into the wild. Meadows, pastures, roadside shoulders, grassy slopes, and the edges of gardens are all common habitats for the yarrow plant in the wild. It can also be successfully grown in flower and herb gardens.

Yarrow has long stems, feathery leaves that grow in pairs, and heads of white flowers that sometimes have a tinge of pink. Its scent is fresh and astringent. Its flowering time is in late summer and it is best cut and dried just as soon as the flower buds open.

SOLVING SKIN PROBLEMS

There are a few skin problems that most of us suffer from at one time or another, and that can be successfully treated with natural methods.

Pimples, blemishes, and blackheads
In the teenage years, and sometimes in the years after for those with oily skin, the main problems are pimples, blemishes, and blackheads. At puberty, hormones run riot, and the imbalance often causes extra sebum to be produced. This causes a build-up in the pores. At first the sebum is white. After about eight hours it hardens, is oxidized by the air, and so it becomes a dreaded blackhead.

If the sebum does not come up to the surface it can form a reddened bump under the skin, and this is what we call a blemish. If the skin is not cleansed properly, this bump can turn into a rather nasty pus-filled pimple. If you have a lot of pimples, then it's acne. This can happen to both boys and girls. Girls are particularly prone just before menstruation when estrogen production is low. Boys experience the condition when they have a rush of male hormones at puberty.

There are, however, some simple ways to counteract the problem. The first thing is always to cleanse the face thoroughly. Use one of the cleansers recommended for oily skins on pages 27-30. If you use soap, use one that is non-alkaline. The medicated soaps sold with the specific purpose of getting rid of pimples may have a sensitizing effect on your skin and are not recommended. Try to avoid touching your face during the day, especially if you have pimples, because you may spread the infection.

Watch your diet. Avoid fatty foods and too many animal fats. Go easy on the tea and coffee. Eat plenty of fresh fruits and vegetables and high-fiber carbohydrate foods such as brown rice and pasta. Drink plenty of water to cleanse your system.

To get rid of blackheads, steam your face once a week with any of the herbs recommended for oily skin. This softens blackheads making it easier to remove them with a cotton ball. Don't force them or dig in your fingernails. You may make things worse.

Another remedy for blackheads is to give your face a warm oil treatment. It might sound

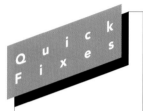

Quick Fixes

• For blackheads and pimples, melt a little honey and spread it over your face. Leave for 15 minutes and rinse off with warm water. This not only softens, but honey is antiseptic and cleansing.
• Use facial scrubs based on oatmeal or cornmeal, and face masks that contain cider vinegar, lemon, or egg white.
• Use an herbal astringent on your face twice a day, letting it dry naturally.

- If you have wrinkles, use rich moisture creams that contain vitamins E and A, and use toners made from chamomile, linden flowers or lemon balm.
- Try a face mask made of 1 egg yolk beaten with 2 tbsp/30 ml milk; or any mask that contains lanolin or mashed bananas.

odd, treating oil with oil, but it again has a softening effect. Have ready a face cloth and a bowl of hot water. Massage a little almond or olive oil into your face. Wring the face cloth out in the hot water and lay it over the affected areas. Let it become cool, wring it out, and lay it on again. Do this several more times until the water begins to get cool. Once again, push out the blackheads with a cotton ball.

Wrinkles and threadveins

Wrinkles are a "problem" that affect us all in the end. The secret is to think about wrinkles early, and keep them at bay for as long as possible. Besides following the cleanse, tone, and moisturize routine, take care of your diet and keep your facial muscles in tone.

Many a time when we were children we were told that if we made an awful face and the wind blew our face would stay in that position. It was just a threat to make us behave, but there is more truth in it than you would think. Wrinkles are caused by our continually making the same expression. This causes the same facial muscles to contract all the time and they eventually become permanently shortened. The skin cannot contract like the muscle and so a dip appears in it which becomes a wrinkle.

It is fascinating to look at children's faces. Unless they are unusually ill or disturbed, their faces are smooth and unlined, and they often look similar to each other. After puberty, we pull faces to match how we think and feel, and our characters and experiences become etched on our faces.

We don't, however, want our experiences to show that much. So we should remember to relax our faces as often as possible. Facial exercises and massage will help to reduce wrinkles, and prevent more from developing. Regular use of nourishing and exfoliating face masks will also help keep your skin soft. (See page 33 for how to apply a face mask.)

Excessive exposure to extremes of weather can cause dry or chapped skin, which in turn lead to wrinkling. Always use a sun block when you are outside, and moisturize your skin well. (See The Effects of the Sun, page 93.)

Threadveins are tiny, broken blood vessels that are visible through the skin, particularly on the face. Drinking too much alcohol can encourage the production of threadveins by depriving the body of B vitamins. Washing with water that is too hot can also lead to the formation of threadveins on delicate facial skin. If you have threadveins, never steam your face.

RECIPE | ASTRINGENT FOR ENLARGED PORES Ⓟ

Chamomile soothes the skin and the vinegar banishes bacteria and dirt. Use this astringent after cleansing the skin.

1 chamomile tea bag

1 cup/250 ml boiling water

2 tbsp/30 ml cider vinegar

1 Place the chamomile tea bag in a pitcher or bowl and pour on the boiling water. Cover and leave to cool.
2 Strain off the liquid and add the cider vinegar.
3 Transfer to a sterilized bottle and store in a refrigerator. Use within one week.

RECIPE | ANTI-BLEMISH NIGHT TREATMENT Ⓟ

The lactic acid in the yogurt combats bacteria, and tea tree oil is a renowned treatment for pimples and blemishes.

2 tbsp/30 ml plain yogurt

1 tsp/5 ml lemon juice

2 drops tea tree oil

1 Mix all the ingredients together in a bowl.
2 Spread the mixture over your face with your fingertips last thing at night.
3 Rinse your face with warm water in the morning.

TEA TREE OIL

Tea tree (*Melaleuca alternifolia*) is a small, shrubby tree native to New South Wales in Australia, that has only recently gained attention in other parts of the world. Its name comes from the fact that its leaves are used as an herbal tea or tisane, but its medicinal properties have been known for centuries by the Aborigines.

Tea tree oil is extracted by steam or water distillation from the leaves and twigs. It is non-toxic and non-irritant, but nevertheless has powerful antibacterial properties. It can be used with great effect to treat oily skin, pimples, acne, rashes, cold sores, and warts. It can also be added to toothpaste.

RECIPE | OATMEAL SCRUB FOR BLACKHEADS Ⓟ

Oatmeal is an excellent skin cleanser, the lemon juice is a mild astringent, and the olive oil softens the blackheads so they leave the skin easily.

2 tbsp fine oatmeal

4 tbsp/60 ml buttermilk or plain yogurt

1 tbsp/15 ml lemon juice

1 tbsp chopped parsley

1 tsp/5 ml olive oil

1 Mix all the ingredients together in a bowl.
2 Spread the paste over your face with your fingertips, taking about five minutes.
3 Rinse off the mixture with tepid water.
4 Splash your face with cold water or with an herbal astringent, and leave to dry naturally.

RECIPE | COMFREY ACNE TREATMENT Ⓟ

This is a freshly scented mask that can be used to cleanse any skin type. It can be on the runny side, so add the egg white a little at a time to achieve the right consistency.

1 tbsp dried comfrey

1 cup/250 ml boiling water

2 tbsp fuller's earth

1 egg white

1 Place the comfrey in a sterilized pitcher or bowl and pour on the boiling water. Cover and leave to cool. Strain.
2 Place the fuller's earth in a bowl and mix in the egg white and 2 tbsp/30 ml of the comfrey infusion.
3 Spread the mixture over your face and leave for 20 minutes.
4 Rinse off the mixture with tepid water.
5 Splash your face with the remainder of the cold comfrey infusion and leave to dry naturally.

RECIPE

ANTI-WRINKLE FACIAL Ⓐ

Rich oils, yeast, honey, and a small amount of cider vinegar to restore the acid balance, will help to control the development of wrinkles. Extra ingredients can be added to suit your particular skin type.

1 tbsp brewer's yeast

1 tbsp/15 ml almond or olive oil

1 tsp/5 ml honey

½ tsp cider vinegar

1 egg yolk or 1 tbsp/15 ml sour cream (dry to normal skin)

1 tbsp/15 ml egg white or plain yogurt (oily skin)

1 Place the brewer's yeast in a bowl and mix in the oil, honey, and vinegar.
2 Beat in the remaining ingredient to suit skin type.
3 Spread the mixture over your face and leave for 20 minutes.
4 Rinse off with warm water. Splash your face with an astringent or cold water. Use a moisturizing cream or lotion to finish the treatment.

RECIPE

EGG AND YEAST FACE MASK Ⓓ Ⓝ

This mask is quite runny, so wrap your hair in a towel. Lay another towel under your head when you apply it.

2 tbsp fresh yeast

1 egg yolk

1 tsp/5 ml olive oil

1 Crumble the yeast into a bowl.
2 Add the egg yolk and beat the two together to form a smooth mixture.
3 Beat in the olive oil, and use immediately.

RECIPE

FRUIT FACE MASKS Ⓐ

The astringent qualities of fresh fruit make it useful for face masks. Use heavy cream for dry or normal skin, egg white for oily.

4 tbsp/60 ml heavy cream or 1 egg white

one of the following: ¼ peach or nectarine, 1 apricot, 3 strawberries, small cube (about 1 in/2.5 cm square) honeydew or watermelon

1 In a bowl, whip the cream until it can stand in a soft peak; or beat the egg white until it begins to froth,
2 Mash the fruit to a puree, having first skinned the peach, nectarine or apricot.
3 Mix the fruit into the cream or egg white, and use immediately.

COMFREY (*Symphytum officinale*)

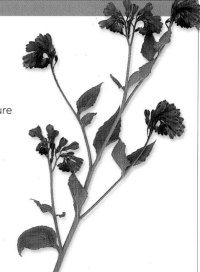

The healing powers of comfrey have been recognized for centuries, and it has long been cultivated in medicinal herb gardens for the healing of wounds and the mending of broken bones. Traditionally, comfrey poultices have been laid on sores, rashes, burns, sprains, and rheumatic or gout-affected joints. Comfrey has many local names which refer to its properties including knit-bone, knit-back, boneset and slippery root. Tea made from the herb was drunk to cure head colds and lung disorders, but internal use is no longer recommended.

Comfrey root and, to a lesser extent, the leaves contain a substance called allantoin that is responsible for the healing properties of the plant. Decoctions made from either part are very emollient, and heal, soothe, and moisturize weathered or chapped skin.

Comfrey grows wild throughout northern Europe and in parts of North America. It can also be successfully grown in damp areas in herb gardens in all temperate parts of the world including Australia and New Zealand. Dried comfrey leaf and root can be found in herbalists and health food stores.

BUTTER FACE MASK Ⓟ

Butter is a good source of vitamin A and so makes an ideal face mask for sensitive, sunburned, or damaged skin.

1 tbsp unsalted butter, softened

1 large strawberry, mashed or 1 in/2.5 cm slice cucumber, chopped and rubbed through sieve (normal to dry skin)

1 tbsp/15 ml lemon juice or 1 egg yolk (dry skin)

1 Beat the butter in a bowl.
2 Beat in the other chosen ingredient, and use immediately.

VITAMIN E FACE MASK Ⓓ

Vitamin E soothes the skin and helps it to repair itself. This mask is good for very dry skin.

1 tbsp/15 ml lanolin

one 100 iu capsule vitamin E

1 Place the lanolin in a bowl.
2 Prick the vitamin E capsule and squeeze the contents into the lanolin. Mix well, and use immediately.

AVOCADO FACE MASK Ⓐ

Choose the recipe you feel most suitable for the way your skin feels on the day. Normal skins will benefit from both recipes.

½ ripe avocado

1 tbsp/15 ml lemon juice (normal to oily skin)

1 egg yolk (normal to dry)

1 tbsp/15 ml plain yogurt

1 tsp/5 ml olive or avocado oil

1 Peel and mash the avocado half in a bowl.
2 Beat in the remaining ingredients, and use immediately.

BANANA FACE MASK Ⓐ

Like avocados, bananas have a rich, creamy texture that enriches your skin when used in a face mask.

½ medium sized banana

1 tsp/5 ml honey

1 tbsp/15 ml plain yogurt (oily skin)

1 tbsp/15 ml heavy cream (normal to dry skin)

1 Peel and mash the banana in a bowl.
2 Beat in the remaining ingredients, and use immediately.

YEAST

Yeast is a natural organism, usually used for raising bread or brewing beer, that can be used in beauty treatments. Fresh yeast is rich and creamy and should be used for dry to normal skins. Brewer's yeast is a nourishing powder that is rich in B vitamins. It can be used for all skin types.

Both yeasts can be successful in the treatment of wrinkles if used regularly. A once-a-week application should be quite sufficient.

MOISTURIZER FOR CHAPPED AND WEATHERED SKIN ◐

This contains marigolds and elderflowers to soothe, and cocoa butter and wheat germ and olive oils to make your skin smooth again. Use it on your face or hands.

2 tbsp dried or 2 heads fresh elderflowers

1 tsp dried marigold or 2 fresh marigold flowers

⅔ cup/150 ml boiling water

1 tbsp/15 ml beeswax

2 tbsp/30 ml cocoa butter

2 tbsp/30 ml wheat germ oil

4 tbsp/60 ml sesame or olive oil

2 tsp/10 ml honey

2 drops lavender oil

1 Place the elderflowers and marigolds in a saucepan with the water. Bring to a boil and simmer for ten minutes. Cool and strain.
2 Place the beeswax, cocoa butter, and oils in the top of a double boiler or in a bowl set in a saucepan of water. Melt gently together on a low heat.
3 Beat in 3 tbsp/45 ml of the flower decoction and the honey.
4 Remove entirely from the heat and beat in the lavender oil. Stir until cool.
5 Transfer the cream to a sterilized pot or jar. Cover when completely cold. Use within two months.

FACE MASK TO TREAT THREADVEINS ◐

Wheat germ, yeast, and vitamin E made into a rich face mask can help to reduce threadveins on the face.

1 egg yolk (for dry to normal skin)

2 tbsp/30 ml egg white (for oily skin)

1 tsp wheat germ

1 tsp brewer's yeast

1 tsp/5 ml wheat germ oil

one 250 iu vitamin E capsule

1 Place the egg yolk or white in a bowl and mix in the wheat germ, yeast, and wheat germ oil.
2 Prick the capsule and squeeze the contents into the bowl. Beat well.
3 Spread the mixture over your face and leave for 20 minutes.
4 Rinse off with warm water. Splash your face with cold water. Use a moisturizer or massage in a small amount of wheat germ oil to finish the treatment.

NECK PACK ◐

This smooths the skin on the neck and helps to reduce any blotchiness. It is like a thick cream in texture, so you need to lie down on towels when applying it. It won't run, but you might like to tie back your hair.

1 egg yolk

1 tbsp brewer's yeast

1 tbsp/15 ml plain yogurt

1 tsp/5 ml wheat germ oil

1 Place the egg yolk in a bowl and beat in the brewer's yeast.
2 Gradually beat in the yogurt, then the wheat germ oil.
3 Apply the neck pack, covering the front of the neck to just behind the ears. Relax for 30 minutes.
4 Rinse off the pack with tepid water then splash your neck with cold water.

NECK CREAM ◐

This will help make the skin on your neck smooth and soft. Use it several times a week, before going to bed.

1 tbsp/15 ml cocoa butter

1 tbsp/15 ml lanolin

2 tbsp/30 ml coconut oil

2 tbsp/30 ml wheat germ oil

2 tbsp/30 ml rosewater, mineral water, or herbal infusion

2-3 drops essential oil

1 Place the cocoa butter, lanolin, and oils in the top of a double boiler or in a bowl set in a saucepan of water. Melt gently together.
2 Remove entirely from the heat and beat in the rosewater, mineral water, or infusion.
3 Beat in the essential oil. Leave to cool, stirring frequently.
4 Transfer to a sterilized pot or jar. Use within three months.

EXERCISE AND MASSAGE

When you exercise the muscles in your body, they become firm and strong. The same applies to the muscles in your face. After exercising, a massage with a base oil plus a few drops of essential oil will relax and invigorate your facial muscles.

Facial exercises

If you devote ten minutes a day to facial exercises you will see positive results in about a month. After that, one session three times a week should be enough. Before you begin, remove any makeup, pat on a toner, and smooth a little moisture cream or base oil—such as almond or jojoba—over your face. Make sure your hands are clean and tie back your hair if it is long. Breathe deeply and try to relax your whole body. Make sure that each side of your face gets equal treatment.

Exercises 1, 11, 12, and 13 require the use of hands. The rest don't and can be done at any time, for example when you are washing the dishes, sitting in front of a computer screen, or waiting at traffic lights.

1 To help relax the muscles, gently stroke your face with your fingertips. Place your hands over your face with your fingertips on your forehead. Gently stroke outwards, over the eyebrows and down over the temples. Do this several times. Run the tips of your fingers lightly down your cheeks, consciously thinking about relaxing the muscles. Lastly, place your fingertips on your chin and stroke up along the line of the cheekbones to your ears. Repeat several times.

ESSENTIAL OILS FOR FACIAL MASSAGE

Cedarwood: for oily skin

Chamomile: soothing and good for sensitive skin and threadveins

Geranium: uplifting, suitable for all skin types, also good for blotches

Lavender: relaxing and refreshing, soothing

Lemon: refreshing and uplifting

Neroli: sensuous, good for threadveins

Rose: expensive and the height of luxury; excellent for the complexion and
   very good for mature skin

Sandalwood: use with geranium for dry skin

Important Before you use an essential oil on your skin, do a patch test to make sure you are not allergic to it (see page 15).

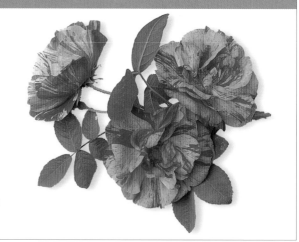

2 Open your eyes very wide for a count of five. Close them and make your eye muscles work as though they are looking down. Hold for five. Repeat.

3 Flare out your nostrils then contract them five times.

4 With your mouth closed, smile wide, hold for two, go into the "oo" position, hold for two. Do this four times.

5 Smile as above and then turn down the corners of your mouth, hold for two each time and do this four times.

6 Open your mouth wide as though you were going to say "ah." Place your tongue behind your bottom teeth. Now try to go into the "oo" position using your lips, but without closing your mouth. Go quickly from one to the other, breathing the sounds "hah, hoo." Do this six times. (You can also try "hah, hee" and "haw, hee" if you enjoy it!)

7 With your lips in the "oo" position, try to force your mouth open while resisting the force with another set of muscles. Hold for ten seconds.

8 Open your eyes wide, raise your eyebrows high and open your mouth wide, keeping your teeth covered with your lips. Hold for 20 seconds if possible.

9 Clench your jaw tightly and push your chin muscles upward. Hold for ten seconds. Push your chin muscles downwards. Hold for ten seconds. Repeat three more times.

10 Fill your mouth with air, blow up your lips and cheeks. Hold for five seconds and let go. Repeat three more times.

11 For smoothing your brow, you need to use your fingertips. To work on frown lines, lay your left finger parallel with your nose with the tip just above your left eyebrow. Place your right fingertip beside your left fingertip, coming down from the top. Push the fingertips past each other, the left one going up and the right one coming down. Reverse the movement and go up and down about ten times. Then place your left finger at the top and your right finger at the bottom and repeat the process.

12 To smoothe away the lines that run across your brow, use the first two fingers of one hand. Place one on the top of your nose and the other toward the top of your forehead. Pull them gently apart so your skin stretches slightly. Rub the forefinger of your other hand along the lines of the wrinkles, five times on each line.

13 Finish by gently stroking your face as in the first instruction.

FACIAL MASSAGE

Massage your face as a continuation of the exercise or as a separate process. Use a plain base oil such as almond, avocado, jojoba, olive, soya, or wheat germ oil. Almond and jojoba are very light oils. Wheat germ is thick and rich, and excellent for dry skins. You can also add 3 drops of essential oil to 1 tbsp/15 ml base oil. See the box on page 48 for suitable oils.

Before you begin, remove any makeup. Make sure your hands are clean and tie back your hair if it is long. Prepare the oil in a small pot then sit and consciously relax for about one minute. Concentrate on giving each side of your face equal treatment.

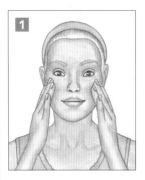
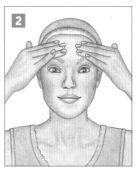
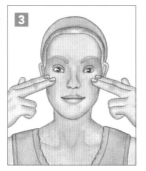
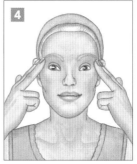
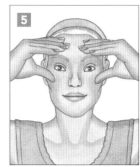

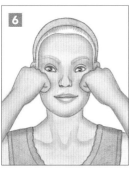
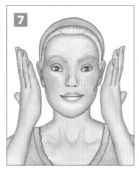
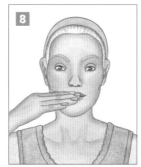
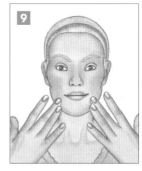
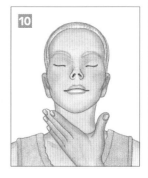

1 Using small, circular movements of your fingertips, lightly spread oil over your face.

2 Place your fingertips above your eyebrows, toward the center of your face. Press gently on and slide your hands outwards to your temples. Repeat, gradually working up toward the hair line.

3 Place the tips of the two longest fingers on each hand just above your eyebrows near the top of your nose. Take them out over the brow line and back under the eye following the line of the top of the cheekbone, then back up the top of the nose to the starting position in a smooth circular movement. Repeat several times.

4 Massage your temples with backwards circular movements of your fingertips.

5 Place your fingers just above the eyebrows and your thumbs under the cheekbones near your nose. Slide your thumbs outwards toward your ears.

6 Make your hands into fists and, using the second joint of your knuckles, gently massage across your cheeks just below the cheekbones.

7 Using the flat of your hand, drum very lightly on your upper cheeks.

8 Place your fingertips on your upper lip and press gently inwards several times.

9 Place the tips of your fingers on your chin. Slide them firmly along the jaw bone toward the ear. Take the fingers off and drum them back down again. Repeat, then slide your fingers in the same direction several times.

10 Stroke your neck in an upward direction. Finish by stroking your face as in exercise 1.

EYES

Look at a person's eyes and you can tell how they are feeling both physically and mentally. Bright, shining eyes with clear, smooth skin around them usually mean good health. Whether you are happy, sad, or worried is shown by the tensions of the various muscles around your eyes. Eyes are a valuable asset, both to the way that you perceive the world and to the face that you present to it. They are well worth looking after.

Eye care

The skin around your eyes is thin and delicate, and needs to be handled with care. Even if you have just bought an expensive eyeshadow or liner, if it causes an allergic reaction, throw it away. If your lids or undereye skin ever become irritated, don't put eye makeup on until the rash has completely cleared. It is far better to have a bare face than sore, puffy eyes. Only use makeup that is designed for eyes or is dual purpose, and make sure that liner pencils are sharpened so that they do not scratch.

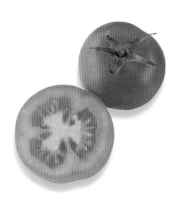

When cleansing your face, use a special eye makeup remover or a gentle facial cleanser. Don't drag a rough tissue across the eye area, but wipe it gently with a cotton ball. When applying a face mask—especially an exfoliator—avoid the area directly around the eyes. Instead, lay damp cotton balls or slices of cucumber over the eyes.

Try to leave your eyebrows as natural as possible. In the past it was fashionable to pluck them out and pencil in a different shape, but eyebrows usually fit the shape of your face and so a little tidying up, if anything, is all that they need. If you have any hairs that are growing out of place and spoiling an otherwise neat line, pluck them out quickly with tweezers. If your brows look dull, rub in a drop of olive oil or use the "Lash and brow conditioner" on page 54.

To keep eyelashes long, lustrous, and in condition, remove all traces of mascara before you go to bed at night. Use the conditioning treatment, or coat them with a little olive oil. If you wear false lashes don't leave them on for too long, or take them off roughly. This can damage the real ones underneath.

To keep eyes healthy eat plenty of foods rich in vitamin A such as carrots, parsley, celery, spinach, peaches, and tomatoes. Eyes also benefit from B vitamins and vitamin C.

Lack of sleep inevitably shows in and around your eyes. Telltale dark rings and puffiness of the undereye tissue are often the result of going to bed late. Other causes are stress, illness, or a sluggish elimination system, which can be helped by drinking lots of water.

Smoke is an irritant to your eyes. Nicotine can also cause a restriction of the blood vessels in the eyes, which may impair your ability to see in the dark. Smoking can also have an adverse effect on your perception of color. Stopping smoking is the simplest solution.

To avoid straining your eyes when you are working, make sure you always have plenty of light directed in the right place. Straining your eyes is not good for long-term vision. It also makes you screw up the surrounding muscles, causing the eventual formation of wrinkles. Continual squinting causes wrinkles, so wear sunglasses in bright weather, especially when you are driving or walking toward the sun.

EYEBRIGHT (*Euphrasia officinalis*)

Eyebright was named not only because of its eye-soothing properties, but because its tiny white, lilac or purple flowers look like small, bright eyes. It has been used medicinally since the fourteenth century. An infusion of eyebright, preferably made with distilled water, makes a safe and soothing eyebath or a compress for tired or puffy eyes.

Eyebright grows wild in northern Europe, northern and western Asia and North America. There are about twenty species altogether.

Eyebright must be planted alongside grass, because it is a semi-parasitic plant that gets part of its nourishment by sending out suckers to the roots of other plants. You can buy dried eyebright from herbalists.

Eye exercises

Keep your eyes in good condition by doing eye exercises that tone and strengthen the muscles.

1 Sit up straight, and consciously relax your facial muscles. Look right ahead.

2 Point your index finger out in front of you, and focus on the tip. Slowly bring it to your nose, keeping your eyes on it. Point it forwards again. Let your eyes follow it, then look at the farthest point you can see. Point outwards again and repeat three more times.

3 Point your right index finger out in front. Focus on the tip of your finger, gradually sweeping it to the right. Facing forwards all the time, follow the finger with your eyes as far as you can. Bring it to the front. Repeat three times, then do the same with your left hand.

4 Look straight ahead and focus on an object in front of you. Turn your head as far to the right as you can while keeping your eyes in the same direction. Bring your head back to the front then move it to the left.

5 With your head level, slowly roll your eyes up and down as far as they will go. Repeat three times.

6 With your lids closed, slowly roll your eyes around in circles, three times in each direction.

• To refresh tired eyes, lie down with one of the following over each eye: a slice of cucumber; cotton balls soaked in an infusion of borage, chamomile, or fennel; a mixture of warm water and milk.

• To reduce puffiness, lie down with one of the following over each eye: cotton balls soaked in witch hazel, or a decoction of peppermint, or rosemary; tea bags, steeped in boiling water, taken out and left until warm. (Spread a thin layer of oil or moisturizer around your eyes first to avoid staining the skin.)

• For dark circles, grate a small potato or cucumber and divide in two. Place each portion between two small squares of muslin, cheesecloth, or an old handkerchief. Use the squares as undereye packs, leaving them on for 20 minutes. Moisturize after using the potato, as it can be astringent. Alternatively, lie down with cotton balls soaked in a decoction of linden flowers over each eye.

• For baggy eyes, paint the skin under your eyes with egg white and let dry naturally before applying makeup.

• For lines around the eyes, lie down with cotton balls soaked in warm oil over each eyes. Leave for 20 minutes. (Choose any of the oils listed on page 48.) Try the massage and eye exercises given on these pages.

RECIPE

CREAM TO SMOOTH LINES AROUND THE EYES Ⓐ

Use this soft-textured cream as an overnight treatment for the delicate skin around the eyes. Smooth it on with your fingertips, using the massage movements from page 50. By morning, it will have been absorbed.

1 tbsp/15 ml cocoa butter

1 tbsp/15 ml lanolin

1 tsp/5 ml wheat germ oil

1 small sprig fresh rosemary or 1 drop rosemary oil

1 Place the cocoa butter, lanolin, and wheat germ oil in the top of a double boiler or in a bowl set in a saucepan of water. If using the sprig of rosemary, add now. Melt the ingredients together, then keep the mixture on a very low heat for ten minutes.
2 If using the rosemary oil, there is no need to keep the mixture on the heat. When the cocoa butter and lanolin have melted, remove entirely from the heat and beat in the essential oil.
3 Remove the rosemary spring, and leave to cool, beating frequently.
4 Transfer to a sterilized pot or jar. Cover when completely cold. Use within two months.

RECIPE

PACK TO TIGHTEN UNDEREYE TISSUE Ⓐ

When you have puffy or tired eyes and the bags are beginning to show, lie down and relax with this undereye pack. Both the rest and the pack will benefit you tremendously.

1 small sprig fresh rosemary

⅓ cup/90 ml boiling water

1 tsp ground almonds

1 tbsp/15 ml egg white

1 Place the rosemary sprig in a pitcher or bowl and pour on the boiling water. Cover and leave to cool. Remove the rosemary sprig. Strain.
2 Place the ground almonds in a bowl. Mix in the egg white and 2 tbsp/30 ml of the rosemary infusion.
3 Dab the mixture under your eyes. Lie down and relax for 15 minutes. Rinse off with warm water and pat dry.
4 Massage the area with almond oil as the egg white can be rather drying.

EYE GEL ⓐ

For a quick, emergency treatment for loose skin under the eyes, try this gel. The protein in the gelatin nourishes the skin beneath the eye, as well as making it smooth and tighter.

1 tsp dried or 1 tbsp fresh chopped eyebright leaves

1 tsp dried or 1 small sprig fresh elderflowers

1¼ cups/275 ml water

1½ tsp powdered gelatin

1 Place the eyebright and elderflowers in a saucepan with the water. Cover, bring to a boil and simmer for 15 minutes. Cool and strain.
2 Place the gelatin in a small saucepan with 4 tbsp/60 ml of the decoction. Leave to soak for ten minutes.
3 Add a further 2 tbsp/30 ml of the decoction. Set the pan on a low heat and melt the gelatin.
4 Transfer the gel to a sterilized pot. Cover when completely cold and solidified. Use within six weeks.

LASH AND BROW CONDITIONER ⓐ

This has the consistency of salad dressing and will separate when left. The sage has darkening qualities when used regularly. The oil will make your brows and lashes smooth and glossy. Use every evening for one month, then once or twice a week.

1 tsp dried sage or 1 tbsp fresh chopped sage

⅔ cup/150 ml water

4 tbsp/60 ml olive oil

1 Place the sage and water in a small saucepan. Bring to a boil and simmer for ten minutes. Cool and strain.
2 Put 2 tbsp/30 ml of the decoction into a small, sterilized bottle or jar.
3 Add the olive oil and shake well. Always shake before use. Use within one month.
4 Massage the mixture into your eyebrows, always ending by stroking the brows in the direction of hair growth. Use a clean mascara brush to apply it to your top and bottom lashes.

MOUTH

A bright smile and sweet breath go a long way toward making a person attractive, so take care of your lips, clean your teeth well, and watch your diet.

The mouth is a special part of your face because the skin on the lips is much more delicate than elsewhere. It has a very thin upper layer of skin cells, making it more vulnerable to extremes of temperature and rough weather. Because lips have no sweat glands, their only protection against the outside world is the saliva produced in the mouth. This is fine at normal temperatures, but continual licking when the weather is very cold or very hot can do more harm than good, and cause the lips to crack. You have to be careful, therefore, that your mouth is adequately protected. Use a sunscreen stick with a high Sun Protection Factor (SPF) when the weather is hot, and a creamy lip balm in cold weather and high winds.

If you don't have a cream lip balm at hand, honey is very effective and a great healer. Melt a tablespoon of honey with a teaspoon of rosewater or mineral water and let it cool. Carry it around with you in a small pot to be used whenever needed.

Teeth

Healthy teeth are usually attractive teeth and there are three easy ways to keep them that way: eat a healthy diet with little or no sugar; clean your teeth regularly, and visit the dentist twice a year for a checkup.

Sugar and refined carbohydrates are notoriously bad for your teeth, causing a buildup of plaque on the enamel. Avoid them as much as possible. The best foods for your teeth are fruit, vegetables, and unrefined carbohydrates such as whole grain bread. To keep your gums massaged and in good shape, eat foods that you have to chew well. If you eat a wide range of natural foods you should have no problem in providing the right vitamins for healthy teeth. They particularly need vitamin D (which helps the body assimilate the calcium teeth need), vitamin C to protect the enamel, and vitamin A for good maintenance.

Many people don't floss their teeth before cleaning with a toothbrush, claiming that it is a messy business or that it takes up too much time. However, most dentists recommend flossing because it can remove awkwardly placed food particles that you may not be able to brush out.

Brushing your teeth not only cleans around, between, and behind them, it also stimulates your gums and keeps them healthy.

Breath

The sweetness of your breath depends on good diet and clean teeth. Fresh, natural foods, as always, will serve you best and it goes without saying that if you have an important date you should watch out for raw garlic and onions!

Mouthwashes help to reinforce the good work done by the toothbrush and also to keep your breath sweet. Strong herbal infusions or decoctions are the simplest mouthwashes. Recommended herbs are marjoram, peppermint, rosemary, sage, and thyme. You can also chew parsley as a quick breath freshener.

HONEY LIP BALM

Honey soothes and repairs cracked lips. It also tastes very good! You can use this lip balm whenever necessary.

1 tbsp/15 ml beeswax

4 tbsp/60 ml almond oil

1 tsp/5 ml honey

For extra soothing qualities add one or all of the following herbs:

1 tsp dried or 1 tbsp fresh chopped marshmallow leaves

1 tsp dried marigold flowers or 2 fresh marigold heads

½ tsp dried or 2 tsp fresh chopped comfrey leaves

1 Place the oil and beeswax in the top of a double boiler or in a bowl set in a saucepan of water. Melt them gently together on a low heat.
2 Remove entirely from the heat and stir in the honey. Stir until the mixture is just warm and transfer to a sterilized pot. Cover when completely cold.
3 If adding the herbs, keep the mixture at simmering point for 15 minutes. Strain into a sterilized pot and add the honey. Stir until cool. Cover when completely cold. Use within three months.

ROSEMARY LIP BALM

Use this firm-textured, green lip balm for chapped or cracked lips.

4 tbsp/60 ml olive oil

1 tbsp/15 ml beeswax

2 tbsp rosemary leaves

2 tbsp/30 ml rosewater

1 Place the oil and beeswax into the top of a double boiler or in a bowl set in a saucepan of water. Melt them gently together on a low heat.
2 Stir in the rosemary and the rosewater.
3 Keep at just below simmering point for 30 minutes.
4 Strain into a sterilized pot or jar. Cover when completely cold. Use within three months.

ROSEMARY MOUTHWASH

Keep this fresh herbal mouthwash in the bathroom ready for use.

2 tsp dried rosemary or 4 rosemary sprigs

4 cloves

2 cups/400 ml mineral water

1 Place the rosemary and cloves in a saucepan with the water. Bring to a boil and simmer for 15 minutes. Cool and strain.
2 Store in a sterilized bottle in the bathroom. To use, dilute it one-to-one with water.

ROSEMARY (*Rosmarinus officinalis*)

The sweet, pungent scent of rosemary has long been associated with cleanliness and the fight against disease. In medieval times, people serving at table in manor houses had to use a rosemary mouthwash so that their breath did not offend the guests, and rosemary leaves were charred with bread and pounded to make a tooth cleaner. Rosemary was burned on open fires to fumigate sickrooms, and hung around the house or put into potpourris to make the air smell sweet. Bunches of rosemary were laid in chests and cupboards among clean linen, and the dried leaves were ground to a powder and rubbed on clothes and gloves. Large branches were sometimes laid over floors so that they would release a sweet scent as they were trodden on.

TEA TREE AND PEPPERMINT MOUTHWASH

Tea tree oil and peppermint will freshen the breath and help keep away bacteria.

1¼ cups/275 ml mineral water

6 drops tea tree oil

6 drops peppermint oil

1 Pour the water into a sterilized bottle.
2 Add the essential oils, cover and shake well.

SALT TOOTH CLEANER

This is a pleasant-tasting tooth mixture. The peppermint freshens the mouth and the tea tree oil combats bacteria.

1 tsp fine sea salt

1 tsp dried sage (optional)

1 tbsp arrowroot

½ tsp bicarbonate of soda

10 drops peppermint oil

5 drops tea tree oil

1 Grind the salt and sage together using a mortar and pestle or a coffee grinder.
2 Combine all the dry ingredients.
3 Mix in the essential oils.
4 Store in a sterilized pot or jar in the bathroom. To use, moisten your toothbrush with cold water and dip it into the powder. Clean your teeth in the usual way. Rinse with cold water. Use within one month.

CHARCOAL AND SAGE TOOTH CLEANER

The idea of using a black powder as a tooth cleaner may sound unusual, but charcoal has a very beneficial effect on teeth. When you finally rinse, your teeth will be sparkling clean and your mouth will taste very fresh.

1 slice whole grain bread

2 tsp dried sage

2 drops peppermint oil

1 Remove the crusts from the bread. Toast the bread until crisp and black on both sides. Leave to cool.
2 Crush the bread into fine crumbs using a mortar and pestle or a coffee grinder.
3 Add the sage and peppermint oil and crush everything together.
4 Keep the mixture in a sterilized pot or jar in the bathroom. To use, moisten your toothbrush with cold water and dip it into the powder. Clean your teeth in the usual way. Rinse with cold water. Use within one month.

SAGE (Salvia officinalis)

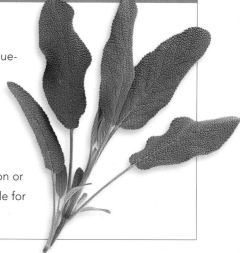

Sage is native to the Mediterranean regions, but now many different varieties are cultivated throughout the temperate area of the world. The most effective type of sage to use to make beauty and medicinal preparations is purple sage (Salvia officinalis purpurea). It has the same tongue-shaped leaves as common sage, but they have a slightly maroon-red tinge. Many people say that the flavor of purple sage is also finer, and so it is also grown for culinary purposes.

All varieties of sage grow easily in a warm, dry spot in any type of soil. The plants will last many years and cuttings are easy to take. If you can't grow it yourself, dried purple sage is often sold in specialist herbs shops. Alternatively, use fresh or dried common sage in the recipes.

Sage has antiseptic properties and has long been known as an effective tooth cleaner. An infusion or decoction of sage makes a good mouthwash and breath freshener, besides being a soothing gargle for sore throats, and an effective cure for bleeding gums.

H A I R

cleanse

condition

color

nourish

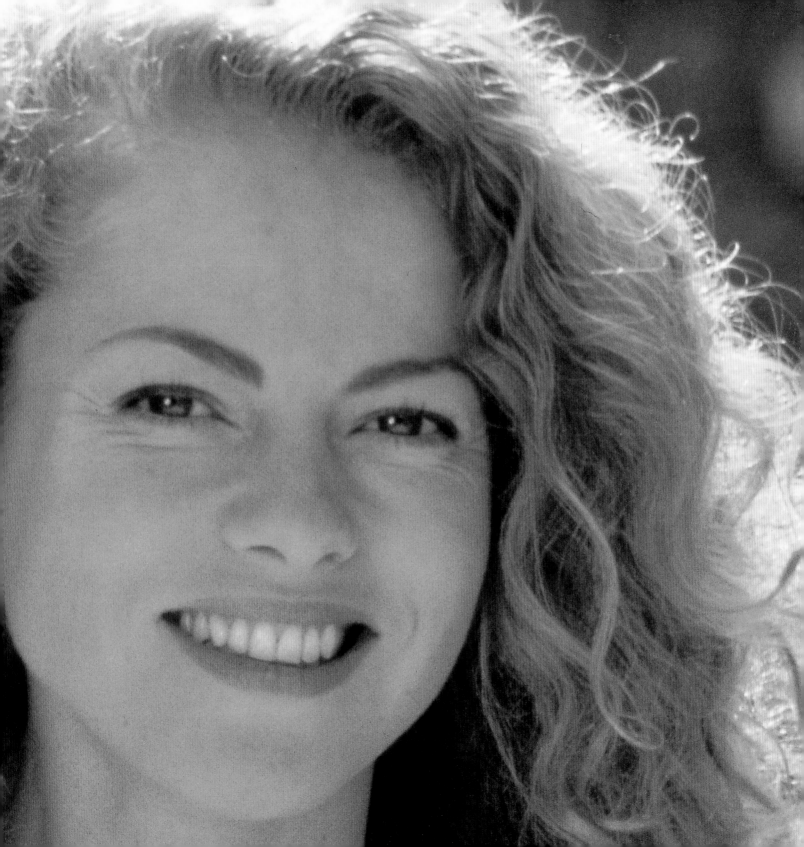

Our hair, like our face, is a part of us that is constantly on show. How a person takes care of their hair, cuts it, and styles it, is ofen a clue to their personality. It is all too easy to give our hair a quick rinse in the shower, a rapid blow dry, and then forget all about it. But hair, like skin, benefits from care and attention.

The type of hair you have, its thickness, color and texture is mainly inherited. The average adult head grows between 90,000 and 150,000 hairs, each of which can survive for between two and ten years. Like your skin, your hair is a reflection of your general health and well-being. It can be affected by diet, stress, illness, and hormonal changes. A healthy head of hair is usually an indication of a healthy mind and body.

Hair is made mostly from a protein called keratin. Each hair begins its formation as a cluster of cells in the lower layers of skin and it pushes upward from an indentation of the skin called a follicle. How thick this follicle is determines the thickness of the hair. As the hair grows it hardens and is fed from tiny blood vessels inside the follicle and lubricated by sebum from the sebaceous glands in the skin beside it. At the same time, it leaves behind more cells that will eventually replace the hair when it falls out.

The average rate of growth for a single hair is about ½ in/13 mm a month, but it can be as much as 1 in/2.5 cm. Because so many hairs are continually replacing themselves, it is quite normal to lose between 50 and 150 hairs a day. It is only when the replacement system fails that hair loss is noticeable.

Each single hair is made up of three separate layers. The soft, inner core, to which the blood vessels deliver the nourishment for the hair, is called the medulla. The middle part, called the cortex, is strong and pliable, and contains the pigment that gives the hair its color. The cortex is actually made up of two parts: the tough paracortex, and the more delicate orthocortex. It is the proportion of one to the other—a factor that is usually inherited—that determines the strength of your hair.

The outer part is called the cuticle. It protects the other layers and consists of overlapping scales. When your hair is in good condition these scales lie flat, reflecting the light and making your hair look smooth and shiny. When your hair is in poor condition the scales stick up in all directions, and your hair will look dull and may be difficult to comb.

Excessive contact with the sun can bleach and dry your hair. Wear a hat in strong sun and condition well at the next wash. Strong winds tangle your hair and can damage the cuticle. Chlorine and salt are both drying, so wash and condition your hair thoroughly after swimming in a pool or in the ocean.

Diet

Diet is important to the condition of your hair, which needs natural oils to stay healthy. Make sure you include nuts, oily fish, sunflower, and olive oils in your diet, especially if your hair is on the dry side. Hair needs an adequate supply of dietary proteins to help it to grow healthily, so include at least one protein meal a day.

CLEANSING

It was once thought that washing your hair too often would destroy its natural oils, but current thinking is that, as long as your hair is in good condition and you use a mild or herbal shampoo, you can wash your hair as often as you want to. Like skin, hair has an acid mantle so it important not to use an alkaline-based shampoo.

Daily brushing cleans your hair of dust, dirt and dead cells from the scalp, and increases the circulation. This in turn encourages new hair growth. Brushing also helps to distribute natural hair oils, and it can be a very relaxing experience.

Tugging gently at your scalp improves the circulation and leaves you feeling refreshed, but it is not advised if you are suffering from a scalp disorder. Starting at the brow line, slide your fingers about 1 in/2.5 cm into you hair. Grasp the hair under your hand at the lowest point and tug gently. Work over your whole scalp in the same way.

Generally, your hair should need only one shampooing. If your hair is very greasy, you may find the shampoo lathers better if you rub it into your dry hair before adding water. You may need to shampoo more than once if you have been to the beach and your hair is full of suntan oil and salt, or if you have used a lot of hairspray or styling mousse since the last wash.

Towel your hair dry and, if possible, let it dry naturally. Using an electric dryer every day will harm your hair, so give your hair the chance to dry naturally on some days. When you do use a dryer, don't hold it too near your head, fit

HERBS FOR HEALTHY HAIR

Herbal infusions make excellent rinses, and small quantities of an infusion can be added to shampoos and conditioners. It is a good idea to make up a large amount of infusion, use a small amount for the shampoo or conditioner, and pour the rest through your hair several times. This way you will save yourself the trouble of making up two preparations, and your hair will get a double herbal treatment.

For normal hair: Chamomile (light hair), elderflowers, fennel, horsetail, nettle, rosemary, sage (dark hair)

For dry or damaged hair: Chamomile (light hair), comfrey, elderflowers, linden flowers, marshmallow, parsley, sage (dark hair)

For oily hair: Lavender, lemon balm, peppermint, rosemary, southernwood, thyme, yarrow

To give body: nettle, rosemary

To give extra shine: cleavers, linden flowers, marigold, nettle, parsley, sage (dark hair)

To tone the scalp: cleavers, fennel, lavender, linden flowers, nettle, rosemary

To improve hair growth: nettle, rosemary, thyme, yarrow

To repair the acid balance: raspberry leaves

To add fragrance: jasmine, lavender, rose, rosemary, thyme, violet

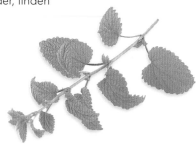

it with a diffuser, and keep the heat low. Heated rollers, curling irons, and crimpers are also very drying to the hair. Don't use them too often and never on wet hair. When your hair is wet, use a comb with round ends and teeth set wide apart. Comb gently so as not to damage the hair.

CONDITIONING

If your hair looks dull, it may be because the scales on the cuticle of your hair are standing up unevenly. A conditioner will help to smooth them down and make your hair look shiny. Conditioners can be applied before washing your hair or after.

A prewash conditioner is worked into the hair, and the hair wrapped in hot towels and left for at least 15 minutes. The conditioning ingredients can then penetrate the hair completely before it is washed.

Afterwash conditioners are rubbed into wet hair after the shampoo has been rinsed out. When using these conditioners, concentrate on the hair ends only and do not massage them into the scalp. An afterwash conditioner can be left on for about five minutes or be washed off once the hair is coated. Instructions for use are given in each of the recipes that follow.

RECIPE · SOAPWORT SHAMPOO Ⓐ

The naturally frothy herb, soapwort, makes a mild and effective hair shampoo that can be used every day without harming your hair. Soapbark can be used in the same way.

1 tbsp crushed soapwort root or soapbark

1 tbsp chosen herb

3 pints/1.5 liters water

1 Place the soapwort root and herb in a saucepan with the water and bring to a boil. Cover and simmer for four minutes.
2 Remove from the heat and leave to cool.
3 Strain, pressing down well.
4 Transfer the decoction to a sterilized bottle and use within one month.
5 To use, wet your hair and rub in about ¾ cup/200 ml of the shampoo. Rinse well with clear water, or with an herbal infusion to match the shampoo.

RECIPE · SIMPLE HERBAL SHAMPOO Ⓐ

This shampoo is a good way to apply the herb that you need to treat your hair, especially if you follow it with a rinse made from the remaining decoction.

⅔ cup/150 ml baby shampoo

1 tbsp dried or 3 tbsp fresh chopped chosen herb

1¼ cups/275 ml water

1 Place the herb in a saucepan with the water and bring to a boil. Cover and simmer for ten minutes. Cool and strain.
2 Pour the baby shampoo into a sterilized bottle.
3 Add ⅓ cup/90 ml of the decoction. Shake well.
4 Shake before each use and use as ordinary shampoo.
5 Rinse well with clear water, then with an herbal rinse. Use within two months.

RECIPE · RICH EGG SHAMPOO Ⓐ

If your hair is very dry, substitute two egg yolks for the whole egg. If it is oily, use one egg white. Eggs make the hair firm and easy to manage.

4 tbsp/60 ml baby shampoo

2 tbsp/30 ml infusion of chosen herb

1 egg, beaten

½ tsp powdered gelatin (optional)

1 Place all the ingredients in a sterilized jar. Cover and shake well.
2 Use the mixture immediately, massaging it into the hair and scalp.
3 Rinse well with luke warm water, then with an herbal rinse.

RECIPE · HERBAL SOAP SHAMPOO Ⓐ

The mixture for this shampoo becomes semi-set and translucent. To use, take a walnut-sized piece and soften it in your hand with warm water before applying to the hair.

1 tsp dried or 1 tbsp fresh chopped nettles, rosemary, or sage

1 quart/1 liter mineral water

4 oz/125 g rich nonalkaline soap

1 Place the herbs and water in a saucepan and bring to a boil. Cover and simmer for 15 minutes.
2 Meanwhile, grate the soap and put it into a large bowl.
3 Strain the decoction immediately onto the soap and beat well until the soap dissolves. Leave to cool.
4 Transfer to a sterilized pot or jar and use as ordinary shampoo. Rinse well with clear water, then with an herbal rinse. Use within two months.

HERBAL PREWASH CONDITIONER Ⓝ Ⓓ

RECIPE

Warm oil mixed with an herbal infusion makes a simple but effective treatment for dry or normal hair.

4 tbsp/60 ml warm herbal infusion to suit hair type

4 tbsp/60 ml warm olive or avocado oil

1 Pour the two ingredients into a bowl and beat together.
2 Massage the mixture into your hair and scalp.
3 Wrap your hair in a hot towel and leave for 30 minutes.
4 Wash out with a mild shampoo.
5 Use a rinse made from the same herb with 1 tbsp/15 ml cider vinegar added.

AVOCADO PREWASH CONDITIONER Ⓐ

RECIPE

Avocados are rich in oils that give a gloss and shine to your hair. If you have greasy hair, cut in half the amount of oil and add 2 tbsp/30 ml extra infusion.

2 medium-sized towels

1 ripe avocado

4 tbsp/60 ml avocado or olive oil

2 tbsp/30 ml infusion of chosen herb

1 Warm the towels on a hot radiator, or place in a dryer for a few minutes.
2 Mash the avocado to a smooth puree.
3 Beat in the oil and the herbal infusion.
4 Massage the mixture well into your hair and scalp.
5 Wrap your hair in a towel and leave for an hour, if possible. Change the towel after 30 minutes to maintain the warmth.
6 Rinse out with warm water, then use a mild herbal shampoo. Follow this by a rinse with warm water, to which you have added 1 tbsp/15 ml cider vinegar.

MAYONNAISE PREWASH CONDITIONER Ⓐ

RECIPE

Egg, oil, and cider vinegar are all excellent hair ingredients. The homemade mayonnaise that you add to your salad could just as easily be used on your hair!

1 egg

¼ tsp salt

½ cup/125 ml olive oil

4 tbsp/60 ml cider vinegar

1 tsp/5 ml honey

1 Place the egg in a bowl with the salt and beat with an electric beater until it begins to get frothy.
2 Gradually beat in half the olive oil.
3 Beat in 1 tbsp/15 ml cider vinegar.
4 Beat in the remaining oil, followed by the remaining cider vinegar, and the honey.
5 Massage the mayonnaise into your hair and scalp.
6 Wrap your hair in a hot towel and leave for 30 minutes.
7 Shampoo the mixture out by running warm water through your hair. Do not use another shampoo.
8 Use an herbal rinse if wished.

Quick Fixes

• If your hair looks very dry, smooth a little oil onto your hands and rub them through your hair to give gloss and body. Avocado and almond oil can be used directly from the bottle. If you use coconut oil, which hardens when it is cool, keep a little in a pot and smear it over your hands to soften it when needed.

PREWASH CONDITIONER WITH EGG Ⓐ

This conditioner froths as warm water is run through it, so you do not need a shampoo. For dry hair, use 1 egg and 2 egg yolks. For very greasy hair, use 2 egg whites and 1 tbsp/15 ml olive oil.

2 eggs

4 tbsp/60 ml warm rosemary infusion

2 tbsp/30 ml olive oil

1 Place all the ingredients in a bowl and beat with an electric beater until the mixture is fluffy.
2 Massage the conditioner into your scalp and hair.
3 Wrap your hair in a hot towel and leave for 30 minutes.
4 Shampoo the mixture out by running warm water through your hair.
5 Use an herbal rinse or add 2 tbsp/30 ml cider vinegar to the rinsing water.

DRY SHAMPOO Ⓐ

When you don't have time for a full hair treatment and you feel your hair becoming dirty or greasy, a dry shampoo is the solution.

1 tbsp fuller's earth

1 tbsp orrisroot powder

1 tbsp arrowroot

10 drops rosemary oil

1 Mix all the ingredients together and store in a sterilized jar for up to two months.
2 Use one third of the mixture for each application. Rub it lightly into your scalp and hair for five to ten minutes. Brush out thoroughly with a soft brush.

ORRISROOT POWDER

Orrisroot powder is the dried and ground root of a species of Iris called *Iris germanica* var. *florentina*, which can be grown successfully as a garden plant in most temperate parts of the world. It is grown commercially around Siena in northern Italy. There, its roots are lifted in the fall and left to dry in huge, fragrant warehouses for three years so they become very hard. These roots are then ground to produce the creamy colored orrisroot powder.

The powder has a delicate violet scent that does not diminish with time, and which is useful for fixing the scents of other ingredients in preparations such as potpourris and in fillings for scented sachets.

HERBAL HAIR TREATMENT

What you will need:

4 tbsp dried or 8 tbsp fresh chopped herb

1 quart/1 liter boiling water

1 Place the herb in a large pitcher and pour on the boiling water. Cover and leave to cool. Strain into a sterilized bottle.

2 Measure out the amount you need for your shampoo and/or conditioner and set aside.

3 When you are ready to use the rinse, reheat the infusion until it is lukewarm.

4 Hold your head over a large bowl and pour the herbal infusion through your hair.

5 Using a small plastic container, pour the infusion through your hair several more times.

6 Gently squeeze out your hair and towel dry.

R E C I P E

EGG AND HONEY AFTERWASH CONDITIONER Ⓐ

After washing out the grease and grime, treat your hair to this nourishing conditioner.

1 egg

1 tsp/5 ml honey

2 tbsp/30 ml olive or avocado oil

4 tbsp/60 ml infusion of chosen herb

1 Using an electric beater, combine the egg with the honey.
2 Beat in the oil, followed by the infusion.
3 After shampooing and rinsing your hair, massage the conditioner into your scalp for five minutes.
4 Rinse out with warm water, to which you have added 1 tbsp/15 ml cider vinegar.

R E C I P E

WARM OIL TREATMENT Ⓝ Ⓓ

Use this as a conditioning treatment for dry to normal hair. If you wish, instead of plain oil, use an oil in which several sprigs of rosemary have been steeped for three weeks.

⅓ cup/90 ml extra virgin olive oil

2-3 medium-sized towels

1 Pour the oil into a heat resistant pitcher or bottle. Warm it by standing it in a saucepan of water on a low heat.
2 Warm the towels on a hot radiator, or place in a dryer for a few minutes.
3 Massage enough of the warm oil to cover your hair into your hair and scalp.
4 Wrap one of the hot towels around your head.
5 Replace the towel as it cools down. Use the other towels in turn while the first warms up again. Try to keep the oil in your hair for 15-30 minutes.
6 To rinse the oil out of your hair, use an herbal shampoo. Rub the shampoo into your hair before adding any water. This will help you to wash away all the excess oil.
7 Rinse with warm water or with an herbal infusion.

R E C I P E

ROSEMARY OIL TREATMENT Ⓐ

Essential oils, added to the "Warm-oil treatment," increase their effect and give your hair a delicious scent.

For dark hair:

⅓ cup/90 ml extra virgin olive oil

15 drops rosemary oil

10 drops lavender oil

5 drops geranium oil

For light hair:

⅓ cup/90 ml extra virgin olive oil

5 drops rosemary oil

10 drops lavender oil

8 drops chamomile oil

For all hair colors:

⅓ cup/90 ml extra virgin olive oil

10 drops rosemary oil

5 drops lavender oil

1 Pour the olive oil into a sterilized jar or bottle.
2 Add the essential oils and shake well.
3 Use as above.
4 To rinse, rub an herbal shampoo into your hair before adding any water.
5 Rinse with warm water or with an herbal infusion.

EGGS

Eggs are nourishing for the skin, relatively cheap to buy and always available, which makes them an excellent ingredient for beauty treatments. The yolk is rich in vitamins and lecithin, a rich moisturizer for dry skin. Egg yolk mixes well with other enriching ingredients.

Egg white is slightly drying and is an excellent skin tightener. Beaten until slightly frothy, it can be used in face masks for dry skin, and in treatments for wrinkled or puffy skin.

COLORING

There are basically two types of hair coloring, chemical and natural. A permanent chemical coloring (one that lasts a long time) has to open up the cuticle (the outer covering of the hair) in order to penetrate the hair. It can damage the cuticle and make your hair very dry. A semi-permanent colorant, that will last for a few weeks does not penetrate so deeply and so causes less damage. A temporary color stays on the surface and goes after one or two washes. Bleaching the hair chemically damages the cortex and also destroys the hair's natural pigments.

Other chemical treatments such as perming and straightening are also harsh on hair because the solutions used break through the cuticle and weaken the hair. Avoid using these processes too often.

When used regularly over a period of time, herbal rinses can bring out the natural highlights in your hair. Use an infusion (or a decoction for a richer effect) of one of the herbs listed in the box to suit your hair color.

For a more intense effect, make herbal hair color treatments. Either make a strong decoction of the herb and mix it to a paste with kaolin powder or fuller's earth; or grind the herb or a mixture of dried herbs to a powder and mix that to a paste with boiling water.

One of the most popular herbs for a coloring treatment is henna (*Lawsonia inermis*). It has been used for centuries in the Near and Far East and has strong coloring properties. The color produced by henna depends partly on where it is grown. (When henna is mixed into a paste, it has a greenish color.) Egyptian and Moroccan hennas give an orange tint, whereas Iranian henna gives a redder color. The length of time that a henna treatment is left on the hair will also influence the final effect. Very often, the shorter the time the treatment is left, the brighter the color. Henna can also be mixed with other ingredients such as chamomile or rhubarb root for light hair; coffee for a dull red, indigo for a very dark brown, and red wine for a rich auburn color.

HERBS FOR HAIR COLORANTS

For light hair: chamomile, great mullein flowers, rhubarb root, St. John's wort

For midbrown hair: marigold, red hibiscus flowers, rosemary, sage, tea

For dark hair: rosemary, sage, southernwood, thyme

For red hair: ginger, juniper berries, marigold, red hibiscus petals, sage

For graying hair: sage

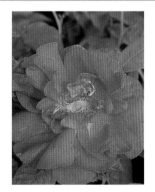

HERBAL HAIR TREATMENT

Before using any coloring all over your hair, do a strand test. Make up a small amount of the treatment and try it on a small strand of inconspicuous hair. Leave it for about 30 minutes, wash it off and decide whether you like the result.

Using henna is a messy business, so spread newspapers all over the floor of the area in which you will be working before you begin.

What you will need:

6 tbsp powdered henna

1 tbsp ground coffee beans, indigo, or powdered herbs

¾ cup/200 ml boiling water (or half red wine, half water)

1 tsp/5 ml cider vinegar to every ¾ cup/200 ml water

large bowl

metal spoon

old towels

newspapers

2 tbsp/30 ml olive oil (normal and dry hair)

hair clips

plastic gloves

kitchen wrap or plastic hat

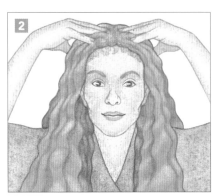

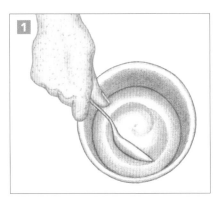

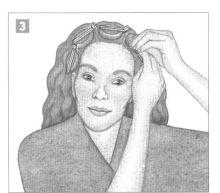

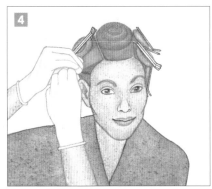

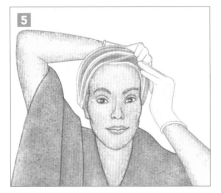

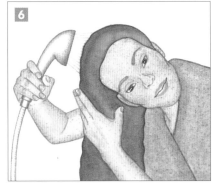

1 Mix the henna and other dry ingredients with boiling water (and wine, if using) to make a thick paste. Add the cider vinegar, then leave the mixture until it is just cool enough to handle.

2 Wrap a towel around your neck and wear an old apron, or place another old towel on your lap. Rub the oil into your hair.

3 Section your hair, using clips.

4 Wearing plastic gloves and working from the center of your head outwards, coat each section of hair with the henna mixture, paying attention to the roots as well as the strands. Pile the strands on top of your head.

5 Wrap your head tightly with kitchen wrap and leave it for the required amount of time. This will vary from 20 minutes to 1½ hours depending on your strand test.

6 Rinse the treatment out of your hair with warm water, easing the strands loose with your fingers. Rinse until the water runs clear. Shampoo and condition as normal.

RECIPE

CHAMOMILE HAIR LIGHTENING TREATMENT Ⓐ

Chamomile will bring out the natural colors in blonde hair, and add brighter highlights to light-brown hair.

2 tbsp dried chamomile flowers

1 cup/250 ml water

1 egg yolk (optional)

kaolin powder

1 Place the chamomile in a saucepan with the water and bring to a boil. Cover and simmer for ten minutes. Strain while still hot.
2 Pour the decoction into a bowl. If using the egg yolk, place in a bowl and gradually beat in the cooled chamomile decoction.
3 Gradually beat in enough kaolin powder to make a paste the consistency of thick cream.
4 Section your dry hair, then cover each section in the chamomile paste.
5 Wrap your hair in kitchen wrap and leave for between 30 minutes and one hour.
6 Rinse the paste out with warm water, then use a chamomile shampoo and rinse.

CHAMOMILE (*Chamaemelum nobile*)

Chamomile gives highlights to blonde and light-brown hair. It also has a highly individual scent in both fresh and dried forms. The plant is indigenous to Britain and Europe, but was taken to North America by early settlers and soon became naturalized. Chamomile is cultivated for medicinal and cosmetic use in England, Belgium, Italy, France, Hungary, and North America.

Since medieval times, chamomile has been grown in Europe in domestic herb gardens, either in beds, or to create a fragrant lawn that gives off a delicious fragrance when walked upon. In prosperous households, a decoction of chamomile and orange peel was put into fingerbowls for use at table.

RECIPE

AUBURN TINT TREATMENT Ⓐ

Use this concentrated sage decoction for a strong, coloring effect.

2 tbsp dried sage leaves

1 cup/250 ml red wine

kaolin powder

1 egg yolk (optional)

1 Place the sage leaves in a sterilized pitcher or bowl.
2 Heat the wine to boiling point and pour over the herb. Cover and leave to cool.
3 Strain the wine into a clean pan and heat it again. Pour it into a bowl.
4 Gradually mix in enough kaolin powder to make a paste the consistency of thick cream. When cool, add the egg yolk.
5 Section your dry hair, then cover each section in the sage paste.
6 Wrap your hair in kitchen wrap and leave for between 30 minutes and one hour.
7 Rinse the paste out with warm water, then use a sage shampoo and rinse.

SAGE DARKENING TREATMENT Ⓐ

Use this to darken brown hair, and to bring out its lowlights. If you wish to make a darker mixture, boil 1 tsp tea leaves with the sage leaves.

1 tbsp dried sage leaves or 2 tbsp fresh chopped

1 cup/250 ml water

1 egg yolk (optional)

kaolin powder

1 Place the sage in a saucepan with the water and bring to a boil. Cover and simmer for ten minutes. Strain while still hot.
2 Pour the decoction into a bowl. If using the egg yolk, place in a bowl and gradually beat in the cooled sage decoction.
3 Gradually beat in enough kaolin powder to make a paste the consistency of thick cream.
4 Section your dry hair, then cover each section in the sage paste.
5 Wrap your hair in kitchen wrap and leave for between 30 minutes and one hour.
6 Rinse the paste out with warm water, then use a sage shampoo and rinse.

RHUBARB ROOT AND CHAMOMILE LIGHTENING TREATMENT Ⓐ

Powdered rhubarb root makes another effective base for a chamomile lightening treatment. The root itself also has lightening qualities.

2 tbsp dried chamomile flowers

2 tbsp dried, powdered rhubarb root

1¼ cups/275 ml boiling water

1 Grind the chamomile flowers to a powder in a coffee grinder.
2 Place them in a bowl with the rhubarb root.
3 Mix to a paste with the boiling water. Leave to cool slightly.
4 Section your dry hair, then cover each section with the hot paste.
5 Wrap your hair in kitchen wrap and leave for between 30 minutes and one hour.
6 Rinse the paste out with warm water, then use a chamomile shampoo and rinse.

CHAMOMILE AND RHUBARB HIGHLIGHTING RINSE Ⓝ Ⓞ

Use this after a lightening treatment to enhance its qualities, or after your regular shampoo for a milder effect.

4 oz/125 g fresh rhubarb

1 tbsp dried chamomile flowers

1 quart/1 liter water

1 tsp borax

1 Finely chop the rhubarb and place it in a saucepan with the chamomile flowers and water. Bring to the boil, then cover and simmer for 20 minutes. Leave until warm.
2 Strain. Add the borax to the decoction.
3 Pour the rinse through wet, washed hair several times. If possible, allow the hair to dry naturally.

DARKENING TREATMENT FOR GRAYING HAIR Ⓐ

If your hair is graying slightly at the roots and temples, try this gently darkening treatment. It will help the gray strands to blend in with the brown. Use the rinse after washing (preferably with a sage shampoo), and massage the root ends of your dry hair daily for a week. After this, use once a week.

For the rinse:

2 tsp dried or 2 tbsp fresh chopped sage

2 tsp tea leaves

1 quart/1 liter water

For the massage:

1 tbsp dried or 3 tbsp fresh chopped sage

2 tsp tea leaves

⅔ cup/150 ml boiling water

2 tbsp/30 ml rum

For the rinse:

1 Place the sage and tea leaves in a saucepan with the water and bring to a boil. Cover and simmer for ten minutes. Strain and use when cool.

For the massage:

1 Place the sage and tea leaves in a bowl and add the boiling water. Cover and leave to cool. Strain.
2 Transfer to a sterilized bottle and add the rum. Shake well. Use within two weeks.

SOLVING HAIR PROBLEMS

One of the most visible—and therefore most annoying—hair problems is dandruff. There are two types of dandruff: one the result of a very oily scalp and the other the result of dryness. The oily form of dandruff has the same basic cause as pimples: an imbalance of hormones that triggers the excess production of sebum. The first thing to do is to think about your diet. Cut down on animal fats, but include small amounts of vegetable oils. Eat plenty of fresh fruits and vegetables, and foods containing B vitamins, and cut down on sugar and salt. While the problem persists, massage your scalp daily with a little cider vinegar scented with a few drops of rosemary or lavender oil. Rinse regularly with an infusion of nettles, rosemary, or sage to which you have added 2 tbsp/30 ml of cider vinegar per 1 cup/250 ml of infusion.

The dry form of dandruff is less common and is caused by an excessively large number of skin cells flaking away, including some of the softer new cells from the deeper layers of skin. This type of dandruff is often related to your general health and state of mind, and can be

LAVENDER OIL

Lavender oil is one of the cheapest, most widely available, and most useful of essential oils. Its fresh, clean scent both relaxes and refreshes, and the oil itself has a particularly soothing effect on the skin. It can be put directly on burns, after they have been held under cold water, on sunburned skin, or insect bites.

Lavender oil is distilled from the lavender plant, *Lavandula vera*, which is grown commercially in many temperate countries of the world, particularly France, England, and Tasmania.

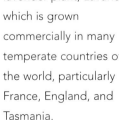

eased by regularly massaging the scalp with a decoction of rosemary. Regular brushing can also help ease the condition.

Dandruff, though, is not as common as you might think. It is normal for small pieces of skin to flake off the scalp as it replaces itself.

Sometimes what we think is skin is actually dried shampoo that has not been rinsed out. Often, good brushing, regular shampooing about twice a week, thorough rinsing, and the occasional hot oil treatment and cider vinegar rinse, are all that is needed to resolve the problem.

RECIPE · TREATMENT FOR OILY HAIR ⊙

Although this smells like a rich fruit cake, it leaves your hair feeling really fresh and clean.

1 tsp dried or 3 tbsp fresh chopped yarrow

1 tsp dried or 1 tbsp fresh rosemary

⅔ cup/150 ml water

3 tbsp/45 ml rum

juice ½ lemon

2 egg whites

1 Place the herbs in a saucepan with the water and bring to a boil. Cover and simmer for ten minutes. Cool and strain.
2 Add the rum and lemon juice, and beat in the egg whites.
3 Rub the mixture into your hair and scalp. Wrap your hair in a hot towel and leave for 30 minutes.
4 Rinse out with warm water, using no other shampoo. Use a yarrow and rosemary rinse if required.

RECIPE · SPLIT-END TREATMENT ℗

Honey and olive oil help to "glue" split ends together. The mixture is rather sticky when you apply it, but leaves your hair feeling soft.

2 tbsp/30 ml clear honey

⅓ cup/90 ml olive oil

1 Place the honey in a bowl and beat in the oil.
2 Massage the mixture into your hair.
3 Wrap your hair in a hot towel and leave for 30 minutes.
4 Rinse out with warm water and use an egg shampoo to follow.
5 Rinse again with warm water, to which you have added 1 tbsp/15 ml cider vinegar.

RECIPE · NETTLE SCALP CONDITIONER Ⓐ

Use this conditioner to make your scalp feel fresh and clean, and to encourage healthy hair growth.

4 oz/125 g nettle tops

2½ cups/575 ml water

2½ cups/575 ml cider vinegar

4 drops rosemary oil (optional)

1 Place the nettles, water and cider vinegar in a saucepan and bring to a boil. Cover and simmer for 30 minutes. Cool and strain.
2 Transfer the decoction to a sterilized bottle, and add the rosemary oil, if using. Shake well. Keep in a cool place and use within one month.
3 Massage a little into the scalp daily and let it dry naturally.

LEMON HAIRSPRAY A

This will help keep your hair in place without the stiffening effect and artificial scent of many commercial hairsprays. The vodka is optional, but it gives the spray a longer shelf-life.

1 lemon

1¼ cups/275 ml water

2 tbsp/30 ml vodka (optional)

1 Chop the whole lemon into pieces and place it in a saucepan with the water. Bring to the boil, then cover and simmer gently for 20 minutes or until the lemon is tender.
2 Strain, pressing down to extract as much liquid as possible. Leave to cool completely.
3 Transfer to a sterilized spray bottle and add the vodka. Keep in a cool place and use within one month.

DANDRUFF-DESTROYING LOTION P

Use this lotion regularly to combat dandruff. Bedtime is probably the best time to apply it, or use it on the days when you have time to let your hair dry naturally.

1 tsp each dried rosemary, sage, and thyme, or 1 tbsp each fresh chopped

2 cups/400 ml water

⅓ cup/90 ml apple juice

2 tbsp/30 ml cider vinegar

1 Place the herbs and water in a saucepan and bring to a boil. Cover and simmer for ten minutes. Cool and strain.
2 Transfer the decoction to a sterilized bottle, and add the apple juice and cider vinegar. Shake well. Use within one week.
3 To use, massage the mixture into your scalp three times a week on the days that you do not wash your hair.

NETTLE (*Urtica dioica*)

Ordinary stinging nettles may seem an unlikely ingredient for hair treatments, but beyond their fierce, outward show, nettles have soothing and cleansing properties. And once picked and dried, or made into an infusion or decoction, their stinging quality is completely neutralized.

Nettles are widespread throughout northern Europe, North America and Australasia. They are so common that you can pick them without having any conservation worries. If you can also encourage a patch of nettles to grow in your garden they will have the added benefit of attracting butterflies.

If possible, pick nettles in spring when the shoots are young, and wear rubber gloves to protect your hands. Always wash nettles well before use.

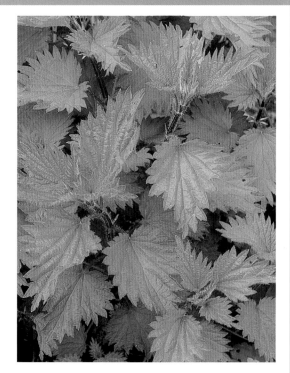

B O D Y

soothe

exfoliate

tone

moisturize

protect

perfume

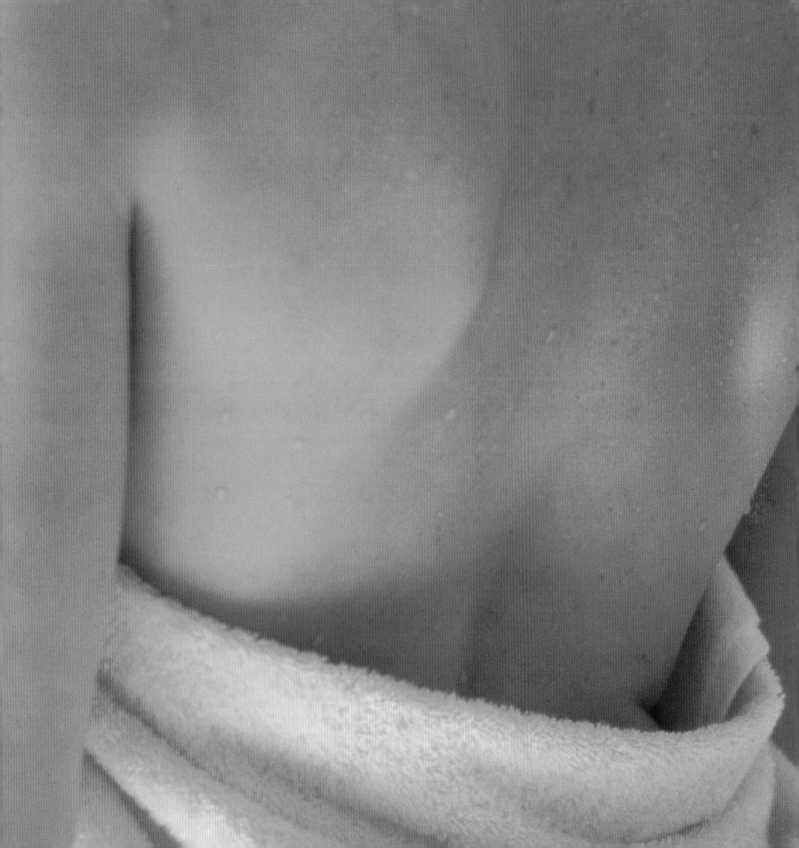

The skin on the body is formed in the same way as facial skin, and has just the same needs, yet it is surprising how often it is neglected. Cleansing, in the form of baths or showers, toning, and moisturizing should figure frequently in your routine, with exfoliating and massage added to the list whenever you feel like extra pampering. Caring for the outside of your body helps to make you feel good inside.

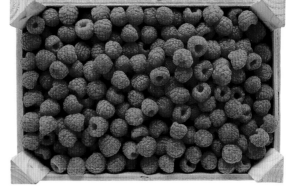

will leave your skin feeling soft and smooth. If you have time, buff your skin with a loofah or a backbrush, or use one of the buffing sachets given below. Towel yourself dry quickly, and apply a body lotion or moisturizer when the skin is still slightly damp.

When you have time, there is nothing quite like a bath. Soaking in warm water relieves tension and tiredness in body and mind. A bath can soothe aching limbs and soak away all the problems of the day. There is even a scientific word for bathing—balneology—which means using water for its curative powers. Taking a bath is an inexpensive luxury that you should make as enjoyable as possible. To do this, follow a few basic guidelines:

• Gather together everything you might need for your bath while the water is running. Use this checklist as a guide: shower cap; large towel or toweling bath robe; essential oils or herbal bath bags to make the bath smell nice; soap or other cleanser; wash cloth or, the ultimate luxury, a natural fiber sponge; a soft

CLEANSING

For a quick cleanse, you can't beat a shower: in the time it takes to run a bath, you can clean your body and wash your hair. An invigorating shower leaves you feeling refreshed, and all the dirt and flakes of dead skin are instantly washed away down the drain.

Even so, just because the process is quick, that doesn't mean you can get away without paying some attention to your skin. Use a mild soap, or a specially formulated shower gel that backbrush; body splash or toner; body lotion or moisturizer.

• The temperature of your bath should be comfortably warm. A bath that is too hot dries your skin and saps your energy. In extreme cases it can put a strain on your heart, since it causes the blood vessels to dilate to cool the body down. If you are going to add herbal bath bags, run the hot tap first to release the herbal essences and then cool the bath down with the cold tap. A very cold bath can be too much of a shock to the system, but one that is pleasantly cool can make you feel great and wakes you up first thing in the morning or cools you down on a hot day.

Soaps and substitutes

Many people swear by soap and water to cleanse the skin. Others claim that soap makes their body feel sticky after use and prefer a substitute. If you are a soap person, make sure that you choose one that is not too alkaline. Alkaline soaps, used frequently, can destroy the skin's natural acid mantle. Use a soap containing glycerine, or one enriched with a natural oil such as wheat germ, vitamin E, or jojoba. Wool fat soaps containing lanolin are also gentle to your skin.

Many good-quality bath gels and bath bubble mixtures act as cleansers in themselves. All you need do, if you use them, is simply use a wash cloth and the bathwater.

Small muslin bags containing ground almonds, cornmeal, or orrisroot plus suitable dried herbs can both scent the bath and be used as gentle cleansers for your skin. There are recipes for these on the following pages.

A plain water bath can be made aromatic, invigorating, sensuous, relaxing, healing, or energizing, depending on what you add to it.

• Adding ⅔ cup/150 ml cider vinegar to the average-sized bath will soften and soothe your skin, and help to conserve the body's acid mantle. To add fragrance and the extra healing powers of herbs, make a herb bath vinegar.

• Milk baths moisturize, nourish, and soften the skin. Simply add about 1¼ cups/275 ml milk to a warm bath. The effect of milk can be increased if it is used in combination with emollient herbs such as elderflower, linden flowers, or chamomile. Make up milk powder and herb bath bags, or infuse the herbs in warm milk for a while.

(Continued on page 80.)

HERBS TO ADD TO YOUR BATH

These herbs will add fragrance and healing properties to the bath water. They can be used alone or in combination to achieve the right balance of effect and scent. Adding loose chopped or dried herbs to the bath is not recommended: the pieces stick to the skin and to the sides of the bath, and block the drain. Use them as an infusion or in bath bags.

HERB	Anti-rheumatic	Aromatic	Astringent	Cleansing	Deodorant	Emollient	Healing	Invigorating	Refreshing	Relaxing	Soothing	Toning
Basil		☐			☐							☐
Bay		☐									☐	
Bergamot		☐									☐	☐
Blackberry leaf								☐				
Borage								☐				
Chamomile				☐			☐			☐	☐	☐
Comfrey						☐	☐				☐	
Elderflower			☐	☐		☐	☐	☐			☐	☐
Elder leaf						☐	☐				☐	
Fennel			☐			☐		☐			☐	☐
Horsetail							☐	☐		☐	☐	
Hyssop	☐	☐						☐		☐	☐	
Lady's mantle						☐					☐	☐
Lavender		☐						☐	☐	☐		☐
Lemon balm		☐						☐	☐		☐	☐
Lemon verbena		☐							☐		☐	☐

HERB	Anti-rheumatic	Aromatic	Astringent	Cleansing	Deodorant	Emollient	Healing	Invigorating	Refreshing	Relaxing	Soothing	Toning
Linden flower				❏		❏				❏	❏	❏
Lovage					❏							
Marigold				❏		❏					❏	❏
Marjoram	❏	❏									❏	
Meadowsweet		❏								❏		
Mint		❏							❏	❏		❏
Mugwort										❏	❏	
Nettle				❏				❏			❏	❏
Pennyroyal		❏						❏	❏			
Peppermint		❏			❏				❏			
Pine needles		❏										
Plaintain leaf							❏					❏
Raspberry leaf			❏							❏		
Rose		❏						❏		❏	❏	❏
Rosemary		❏						❏			❏	❏
Sage		❏	❏	❏				❏				❏
Thyme		❏		❏						❏	❏	
Valerian										❏		
Vervain										❏		

- Salt baths are healing and soothing for the skin. Use a pure sea salt and add about 4 tbsp to the average bath.

- Epsom salts in the bath ease aching limbs and draw toxins from the body. They can reduce stress and help you relax. Dissolve about 1 cup/250 g in 1 quart/1 liter boiling water and add to an average sized bath. Do not use soap in an Epsom salts bath as it stops them working as they should.

DEODORIZING

Sweating is a natural function that performs the important functions of getting rid of waste products and keeping the body at the correct temperature. Even in cold weather, the average person produces about 1 quart/1 liter of sweat every day.

When sweat first arrives on the surface of the body it is colorless and almost odorless. The smell only begins to intensify when it has been around for a while. The smell of fresh sweat is a well-known sexual stimulant, so we shouldn't eliminate it altogether.

If your skin is clean, the smell will develop far slower than if your skin is unwashed, so the first antidote is to bathe or shower once a day. The second is to pay attention to your diet. Eat plenty of fresh fruits, vegetables and whole grains, not too much fat, and a plain yogurt once a day.

If you follow these two principles you will probably find that, for most of the time, all you need is talcum powder under your arms. If there are times when you need extra help, use strong decoctions or infusions of lovage or basil. Paint them all over or just under your arms, and let dry naturally.

If you would rather buy commercial products then use only deodorants. An antiperspirant stops you sweating altogether and this is not good for you.

LOVAGE (*Levisticum officinale*)

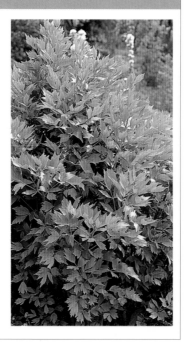

Lovage is related to parsley and has a pungent, celerylike scent and flavor. It originated in the Mediterranean region, but now grows wild throughout most of Europe and in western Asia and North America. It can be grown successfully in herb gardens in temperate climates. It has large, shiny, toothed leaves and small umbrellalike heads of yellow flowers.

In medicine, lovage has been used for digestive complaints, skin problems, menstrual irregularities, and fever. Its antimicrobial, antiseptic, and cleansing properties make it an excellent deodorant. Both the root and the leaves can be used for this purpose.

R E C I P E ## MILK AND HONEY BATH Ⓐ

Milk baths are softening to the skin and feel very luxurious. Use the mixture right away.

4 tbsp/60 ml honey

1 quart/1 liter boiling water

6 tbsp dried milk powder

1 Place the honey in a bowl or large pitcher and pour on the boiling water. Stir until the honey has dissolved. Leave to cool.
2 Place the milk powder in a bowl and gradually mix in the honey water.
3 Add the milk mixture to a warm bath, swishing it about so the milk powder dissolves completely.

R E C I P E ## MILK AND ELDERFLOWER BATH Ⓐ

This has a very softening and soothing effect on the skin. Chamomile or linden flowers may be used instead of elderflowers. Use the mixture right away.

2 tbsp dried elderflowers

1 quart/1 liter boiling water

2 tbsp/30 ml honey

6 tbsp dried milk powder

1 Place the elderflowers in a pitcher or bowl and pour on the boiling water. Add the honey and stir until dissolved. Cover and leave to cool. Strain.
2 Place the milk powder in a bowl and gradually mix in the strained infusion.
3 Add the milk mixture to a warm bath, swishing it about so the milk powder dissolves completely.

R E C I P E ## GRAIN EXTRACT BATH Ⓐ

Grains soften, cleanse and heal the skin. The lavender is relaxing and reviving; the bay relieves aching muscles. Both herbs have a pleasant scent, but they can be omitted or substituted with other herbs if wished.

4 tbsp bran

4 tbsp barley (preferably with the outer skin still on)

4 tbsp brown rice

2 tsp bicarbonate of soda

½ oz lavender flowers

4 bay leaves

3 pints/1.5 liters water

1 Place all the ingredients in a saucepan and bring to a boil. Cover and simmer for 30 minutes. Strain.
2 Add the liquid to a warm bath right away.

R E C I P E ## HERBAL BATH EXTRACT Ⓐ

This works best when the strongly scented herbs or leaves are used singly.

Choose one of the following herbs:

4 tbsp dried or 8 tbsp fresh lavender flowers

4 tbsp dried or 8 tbsp fresh rosemary leaves

6 tbsp fresh, young pine needles

4 tbsp dried or 8 tbsp fresh chamomile flowers

4 tbsp dried elderflowers or 3 fresh elderflower heads

4 tbsp dried or 8 tbsp fresh hyssop leaves and flowers

Plus:

2½ cups/575 ml brandy

⅓ cup/90 ml rose or orange flower water

10 drops of appropriate essential oil (i.e. lavender oil for lavender flowers, rosemary for rosemary leaves.)

1 Place your chosen herb in a sterilized bottle that holds 3 cups/725 ml or slightly more. Pour in the brandy. Seal the top and shake gently.
2 Leave the bottle in a warm place for one week, shaking every day.
3 Strain off the infusion through coffee filter paper, pressing down gently on the herb to extract as much of its scent and properties as possible.
4 Add the rosewater or orange flower water.
5 Rebottle the liquid. Add the appropriate essential oil and shake well. Shake before use. Use 4 tbsp/60 ml per bath. Use within four months.

GROUND ALMOND SOAP Ⓐ

Ground almonds both cleanse and soften. If you are allergic to soap, or if soap makes your skin feel dry or sticky, this is the ideal substitute. It is suitable for all skin types.

2 tbsp ground almonds

2 tbsp fuller's earth

½ tsp borax

1 tbsp/15 ml almond, olive, or sunflower oil

1 Place the ground almonds, fuller's earth, and borax in a bowl.
2 Mix in the almond oil. The mixture should be the texture of very stiff modeling clay.
3 Transfer to a small, sterilized pot and cover.
4 Keep in the bathroom and use as a soap substitute, moistening a knob in the palm of your hand with water until you can rub it over your skin. Use within one month.

HERBAL LIQUID SOAP SUBSTITUTE Ⓐ

This liquid soap substitute is very effective when used in the shower. Essential oils may be added with the almond or olive oil. Choose relaxing or reviving scents to suit your mood.

1 tbsp chamomile, elderflower, or linden flowers

⅓ cup/90 ml milk

½ egg, beaten

4 tbsp/60 ml almond or olive oil

1 tbsp/15 ml baby shampoo

1 tsp/5 ml honey

1 tbsp/15 ml vodka

1 Infuse the herb in the milk for three hours. Strain.
2 Beat the egg and oil together until they are smooth. Gradually beat in the shampoo, honey, vodka, and finally the milk.
3 Transfer the mixture to a sterilized jar and cover. Store in a refrigerator and use within one week. Shake well before use.
4 Use in the shower as ordinary soap, using warm water to prevent the egg from setting.

HERBAL BATH VINEGAR (SLOW METHOD) Ⓐ

Herbal bath vinegars restore the skin's acid balance. Add 1¼ cups/275 ml to a bath of warm water.

6 tbsp dried or 12 tbsp fresh chopped herb(s) of choice

2½ cups/575 ml good quality, light-colored cider vinegar

up to 2½ cups/575 ml mineral water

1 Place the herbs in a 1 quart/1 liter sterilized glass bottle and pour in the vinegar. Cover and leave on a warm, sunny windowsill for three weeks. Shake the bottle every day.
2 Strain off the vinegar through coffee filter paper, pressing down hard on the herbs.
3 Measure the vinegar and add an equal volume of mineral water.
4 Bottle and leave for one week before use. Use within four months.

HERBAL BATH VINEGAR (FAST METHOD) Ⓐ

This bath vinegar is quicker to make and can be used immediately, but it doesn't have so fine a scent. Use it in the same way as the previous recipe.

6 tbsp dried or 12 tbsp fresh chopped herb(s) of choice

2½ cups/575 ml good quality, light colored cider vinegar

2½ cups/575 ml mineral water

1 Place the herbs in a bowl or large pitcher.
2 Place the vinegar and mineral water in a saucepan and bring to a boil.
3 Pour the hot mixture over the herbs. Cover the bowl with a lid or kitchen wrap and leave for 12 hours.
4 Strain through coffee filter paper, pressing down hard.
5 Transfer to a sterilized bottle and use within two months.

SCENTED BATH VINEGAR Ⓐ

This bath vinegar is scented with soothing essential oils. Turn to pages 98-99 for more information on essential oils

1¼ cups/275 ml cider vinegar

jojoba oil

selection of essential oils

1 Pour the cider vinegar into a bottle and add 2 tsp/10 ml jojoba oil.
2 Add up to 40 drops essential oil in the proportions that you have worked out following the instructions on page 98. Cover and shake well.
3 Sniff to test. Correct, if necessary, adding only one extra drop of oil at a time. Add ⅔ cup/150 ml to an average-sized bath. Use within two months.

LOVAGE DEODORANT Ⓐ

This is an effective deodorant that allows the body to sweat naturally, but eliminates unpleasant odors.

1 tbsp dried or 2 tbsp fresh chopped lovage leaves, or 1 tbsp dried chopped lovage root

2½ cups/575 ml water

1 Place the lovage leaves or root in a saucepan with the water and bring to a boil. Cover and simmer for five minutes.
2 Cool completely and strain into a sterilized jar. Store in a cool place and use within one week.
3 To use, soak a cotton ball in the liquid. Wipe it over your body and leave to dry naturally.

EMOLLIENT BATH MIXTURE Ⓐ

This bath mixture leaves your skin soft and scented. You can change the essential oils to suit your mood.

4 oz/125 g pure sea salt

2 tbsp/30 ml cocoa butter, finely grated

10 drops lavender oil

5 drops neroli oil

1 tsp/5 ml base oil

2 tsp/10 ml honey

1 Place the salt and cocoa butter in a bowl and mix well.
2 Add the essential oils, base oil, and honey. Mix well again.
3 Transfer to a sterilized, dark glass container. Use within one month.
4 To use, add 1 tbsp/15 ml of the mixture to an average-sized bath, and swish it about in the water.

TALCUM POWDER Ⓐ

This makes a fine, soft powder that you can scent with the essential oil of your choice.

6 tbsp unscented talcum powder

6 tbsp rice flour or corn flour

2 tsp boric acid powder

1 tbsp orrisroot powder

total of 1 tsp/5 ml essential oil, made up of a single oil or a blend

1 Combine the dry ingredients in a bowl.
2 Add the essential oil and rub it in with your fingertips until it has completely dispersed, and the mixture feels dry.
3 Sieve the powder twice.
4 Pack the powder into a box and leave it for three days for the scent to mature. It will then keep for up to six months.
5 Apply the powder with a large dusting puff.

Recipes for Bath Bags

Each of the bath bag recipes given below will fill eight to ten muslin bags, so it makes sense to make several at a time. To use, hang the bag over the hot tap and let it dangle in the running water. Add cold water to bring the bath to a comfortable temperature. When the bath is full, swish the bag about in the water and squeeze it several times. Leave it in when you have your bath. You can also use bath bags instead of soap: simply rub one gently over your body while you are in the bath.

Dried milk powder, fine oatmeal, ground almonds, cornmeal, or orrisroot powder can be added to the bags.

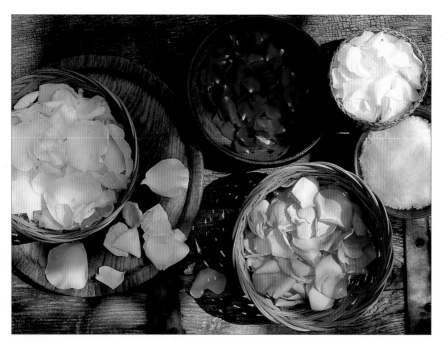

RECIPE

Rose, Lavender, and Almond ⓐ

This mixture is sweetly scented and luxurious.

2 tbsp dried rose petals
3 tbsp dried lavender flowers
4 oz/125 g ground almonds

RECIPE

Chamomile, Linden Flower, and Almond ⓐ

These bath bags are gently emollient on the skin, and relaxing for mind and body.

2 tbsp dried chamomile flowers
2 tbsp dried linden flowers
4 oz/125 g ground almonds

RECIPE

Rosemary, Lemon Verbena, and Cornmeal ⓐ

These bath bags will revive a tired body and a tired mind.

2 tbsp dried rosemary leaves
1 tbsp dried lemon verbena leaves
4 oz/125 g cornmeal

RECIPE

Peppermint, Lovage, and Cornmeal ⓐ

This combination has a refreshing scent and is also a natural deodorant.

4 tbsp dried peppermint leaves
1 tbsp dried lovage root
4 oz/125 g cornmeal

HERBAL BATH BAGS

What you will need:

a piece of muslin, cheesecloth, or thin cotton
3½ x 9½ in/9 x 24 cm.

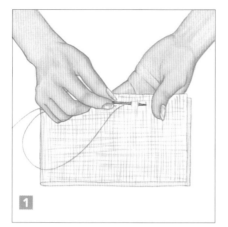

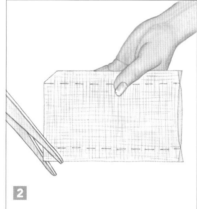

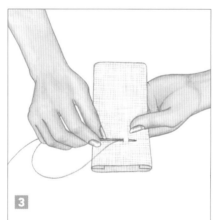

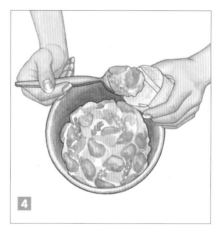

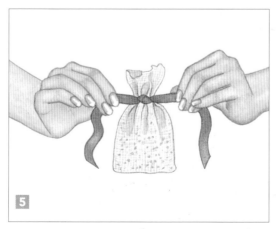

1 Fold the material in half and sew up the long sides, leaving a ½ in/1 cm seam.
2 Clip the corners and turn the bag inside out.
3 Run a gathering stitch around the top of the bag about 1½ in/4 cm from the edge.
4 Fill the bag with your chosen herbal mixture.
5 Pull up the gathers and secure them. Tie the bags at the top with a long piece of string (or ribbon if they are to be a gift). Knot the top to make a loop. The bags will keep unused for up to four months, but should be used only once.

BATH OILS

In these recipes, fragrant essential oils are added to 4 tbsp/60 ml of base oil. The most suitable base oil for the purpose is Turkey Red oil, a castor oil that has been treated to help it disperse in water. If this is unobtainable, use one of the lighter plant-based oils such as almond, jojoba, or even an ordinary sunflower oil. The base oil serves to disperse the essential oils and nourish the skin. As with herbs, choose essential oils for their properties and fragrance.

Add about 1 tbsp/15 ml scented oil to the bath when the water is the correct temperature. Swish the water around to disperse the oil. Once in the bath, gently massage your skin underwater with a sponge.

To make a bath oil, pour the base oil into a dark glass bottle. Add the essential oils, cover and shake well. Leave for two weeks for the scents to blend and mature. Shake before use.

SANDALWOOD OIL

Sandalwood oil is extracted by water or steam distillation from the roots and heartwood of the sandalwood tree (*Santalum album*). The tree—a small evergreen, native to tropical Asia—must be thirty years old before it is ready for the production of the oil. Today, most sandalwood oil comes from India, although some is produced in Europe and the United States.

The properties of sandalwood and its oil have been known for at least 4,000 years. Its scent is warm, sweet, and woody, and it is associated with relaxation and self-expression.

RECIPE

Alcohol-based Bath Oil Ⓐ

Spirits such as vodka or brandy will help to distribute the oil.

⅓ cup/90 ml castor oil

4 tbsp/60 ml vodka

10 drops essential oil(s) of choice

1 Pour the oil and vodka into a sterilized bottle and shake them together.
2 Add the essential oil(s) and shake again. Leave for two weeks for the scents to blend and mature.
3 Add 2 tbsp/30 ml to a average-sized bath, and swish it about in the water.

RECIPE

Shampoo-based Bath Oil Ⓐ

A mild baby shampoo is another efficient carrier of essential oils and base oil.

½ cup/125 ml almond, corn, or sunflower oil

4 tbsp/60 ml baby shampoo

10 drops essential oil(s) of choice

1 Pour the oil into a sterilized bottle.
2 Add the shampoo and shake well.
3 Add the oil and shake again. Leave for two weeks for the scents to blend and mature.
4 Add 2 tbsp/30 ml to an average-sized bath, and swish it about in the water.

RECIPE

Relaxing Bath Oil Ⓐ

Sweet, relaxing scents are given a touch of freshness with oils of lemon and pine.

4 tbsp/60 ml base oil

12 drops sandalwood oil

8 drops orange oil

4 drops rose oil

2 drops pine oil

2 drops lemon oil

Revitalizing Bath Oil

Geranium oil is well known for restoring and revitalizing the spirit, lemon verbena relieves stress, and clary sage brings a touch of happiness.

4 tbsp/60 ml base oil

12 drops geranium oil

6 drops sandalwood oil

4 drops lemon verbena oil

2 drops clary sage oil

R E C I P E

Sensuous Bath Oil

This is a very simple combination. Warm, relaxing orange complements the rich, floral scent of jasmine.

4 tbsp/60 ml base oil

20 drops jasmine oil

8 drops orange oil

JASMINE OIL

Jasmine (*Jasminum officinalis*) is a shrubby evergreen vine with bright green leaves and highly fragrant, star-shaped white flowers. It is native to China, northern India, and West Asia, and is now also cultivated around the Mediterranean.

Jasmine oil has a rich, warm, floral scent with a slightly tea-like undertone. It is frequently used to scent soaps, cosmetics, and perfumes. The scent is said to bring about feelings of confidence, optimism, and the courage to face forthcoming events.

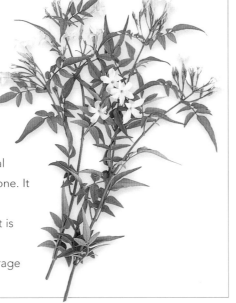

ROSE OIL

The essential oil of the rose has been associated with female sexuality and beauty since classical times. Its scent is uplifting, relaxing, and soothing, besides having a reputation for being an aphrodisiac. Rose oil is an ingredient in many classic perfumes.

Natural rose oil is the most expensive of all the essential oils, but a little goes a very long way. The best is Bulgarian Rose Otto, which is distilled from the fresh petals of the ancient damask rose, *Rosa damascena*. Slightly less expensive is rose absolute, which is produced by solvent extraction in France, Italy and China.

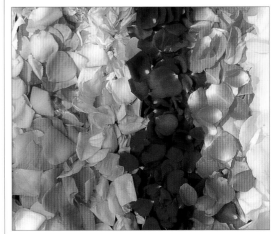

R E C I P E

Happiness Bath Oil

A bath oil to give you a feeling of inner warmth and happiness.

4 tbsp/60 ml base oil

10 drops sandalwood oil

5 drops jasmine oil

5 drops rose oil

5 drops bergamot oil

BODY TREATMENT

If you have an afternoon to spare, try giving yourself a body treatment. The recipes below will exfoliate and moisturize. To use a body treatment, you need a warm room, several old towels to stand and sit on, and a shower or bath nearby.

What you will need:

old towels

prepared body treatment

moisturizer

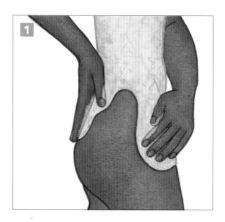

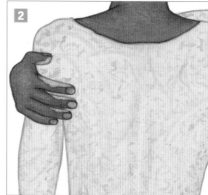

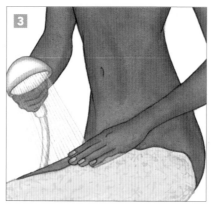

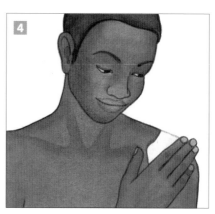

1 Massage the body treatment into every part of your body, avoiding the tender parts such as nipples and genitals. (Better still, get a partner to do it for you!)
2 Leave the body treatment on for 15 minutes, massaging gently.
3 Rinse off the treatment with warm water.
4 Pat dry, and apply moisturizer when the skin is still slightly damp.

EXFOLIATING

The skin on your body, like the skin on your face, needs occasional encouragement to help it get rid of unwanted dead cells. The process is called exfoliation, and it helps the skin to stay soft and smooth. A simple way to exfoliate the skin is to buff it very gently when you are in the bath or shower. Use a loofah or a hemp bath mitt, or make up one of the buffing sachets from the recipes opposite.

To make a buffing sachet, follow the instructions for making "Herbal bath bags" on page 85. Fill the bag with your chosen mixture and sew up the open side.

Salt Buffing Sachet ⓐ

Rubbing your body gently with salt will remove hardened layers of dead tissue.

2 tbsp coarse sea salt

1 tsp bicarbonate of soda

1 tbsp dried elderflower or linden flowers (optional)

RECIPE

Bran Buffing Sachet ⓐ

Bran is softening and healing to the skin.

1 tbsp bran

2 tsp sea salt

RECIPE

Oatmeal and Almond Buffing Sachet ⓐ

Oatmeal cleanses, and the almonds moisturize and give a soft sheen to your skin

2 tbsp oatmeal

2 tbsp ground almonds

SEA SALT

Sea salt is produced by the evaporation of sea water. It contains about 97 percent sodium chloride plus trace minerals that include magnesium, calcium, iron, and zinc.

Table salt is highly refined to remove many of these trace minerals, and magnesium carbonate is added to coat the crystals to make them "free running." Natural sea salt is, therefore, the best to use in beauty preparations.

RECIPE

SALT AND OIL BODY RUB ⓐ

This treatment softens the skin, gets rid of dead cells and improves the circulation.

2 tbsp fine sea salt

2 tbsp/30 ml cider vinegar or lemon juice

½ cup/125 ml olive, safflower, or sunflower oil

1 Moisten the sea salt with the cider vinegar or lemon juice.
2 Standing in the bath in a warm bathroom, rub yourself all over with the oil.
3 Gently massage in the salt, paying particular attention to areas of hard skin such as the knees and elbows. Continue for 15 minutes.
4 Run a warm bath and massage the oil and salt off your skin.

RECIPE

ELBOW SOFTENER ⓓ

Use this twice a day and the skin on your elbows will soften within a week. After that, a weekly treatment should be enough. This is about one week's supply.

4 tbsp/60 ml olive oil

juice 1 lemon

1 tbsp/15 ml honey

1 Pour the ingredients into a sterilized jar, cover, and shake vigorously. Shake well before use.
2 Massage a little into each elbow for about two minutes. Rinse off, pat dry, and moisturize.

RECIPE — BANANA BODY TREATMENT Ⓐ

Bananas are an excellent ingredient for skin care, being emollient but not greasy.

2 bananas

2 tbsp/30 ml olive oil

2 tbsp fine sea salt

2 tbsp ground almonds

juice ½ lemon

2 tbsp/30 ml rosewater or herbal infusion

1 Peel and mash the banana in a bowl.
2 Beat in the oil.
3 Mix in the salt and ground almonds.
4 Beat in the lemon juice and rosewater or herbal infusion.
5 Use within two hours.

RECIPE — RICH EGG BODY TREATMENT Ⓐ

This is a deliciously runny treatment, so stand on plenty of old towels, or get into the shower to apply it. The treatment will moisturize as well as exfoliate.

4 eggs

4 tbsp ground almonds

1 tsp sea salt

2 tbsp/30 ml almond or olive oil (omit if you have oily skin)

juice 1 lemon

1 Beat the eggs together in a bowl.
2 Place the almonds and salt in a second bowl and stir in the oil, eggs, and lemon juice.
3 Use immediately.

RECIPE — OATMEAL AND BUTTERMILK BODY TREATMENT Ⓐ

This is one of the easiest of body treatments to make. If buttermilk is unavailable, use a plain yogurt, or whole milk.

6 tbsp fine oatmeal

¾ cup/175 ml buttermilk or plain yogurt

1 Place the oatmeal in a bowl.
2 Gradually mix in the buttermilk.
3 Leave to stand for 30 minutes before using, so that the oatmeal has time to swell.

RECIPE — AVOCADO BODY TREATMENT Ⓐ

A rich, creamy textured treatment, pale green in color.

1 ripe avocado

2 tbsp fine sea salt

2 tbsp fine oatmeal

2 tbsp/30 ml avocado or olive oil

juice 1 lemon

2 tbsp/30 ml rosewater or infusion of elderflower, linden flowers, or chamomile

1 Peel and mash the avocado in a bowl.
2 Beat in the salt and oatmeal.
3 Add the oil, then the lemon juice and rosewater or herbal infusion. Beat well.
4 Use immediately.

BANANA

Bananas are rich in A and B vitamins and protein, and have a naturally emollient effect on the skin without being oily. As they rarely trigger allergic reactions, bananas are an excellent moisturizer for all skin types.

Eating bananas not only provides you with vitamins and the mineral potassium, but also helps to rid the system of toxins and excess sodium.

HUNGARY WATER Ⓐ

Use this water as a body splash or cologne.

1½ cups/275 ml vodka

3 tbsp dried or 6 tbsp fresh rosemary leaves

1 tbsp dried or 2 tbsp fresh chopped lemon balm leaves

1 fresh mint sprig (if unavailable, omit the mint as the dried herb doesn't have a pleasant scent)

4 thinly pared strips lemon peel

⅓ cup/90 ml rosewater

⅓ cup/90 ml orange flower water

1 Pour the vodka into a jar.
2 Add the herbs, cover tightly and shake.
3 Leave in a warm place for three weeks, shaking every day.
4 Strain and add the rosewater and orange flower water.
5 Transfer to a sterilized bottle and keep in a cool place. Use within six months.

HUNGARY WATER

The first recipe for an alcohol-based perfume was written in 1370. It was for "Elizabeth, Queen of Hungary's Water," which eventually became Hungary water. It is said that the cologne was used by the seventy-two-year-old Queen as a beauty treatment, and so enhanced her looks that she received a proposal of marriage from the King of Poland. She refused him, however, on account of her love for "the Lord Jesus Christ," from one of whose angels she claimed the recipe had come!

COLOGNE Ⓐ

This cologne is scented with essential oils. Turn to pages 98-99 for a list of oils and hints for using them. To make a light toilet water to match this cologne, use half vodka and half distilled water as a base.

½ cup/125 ml vodka

⅔ cup/150 ml dark glass bottle

jojoba oil

selection of essential oils

1 Pour the vodka into the bottle and add 2 tsp/10 ml jojoba oil.
2 Add up to 40 drops essential oil in the proportions that you have worked out following the instructions on page 98. Cover and shake well.
3 Sniff to test. Correct, if necessary, adding only one extra drop of oil at a time. Use within six months.

HERBAL BODY TONER Ⓐ

Refreshing herbs make good body toners. Use an essential oil to match the herb. If using nettles, use peppermint or rosemary oil. Omit the glycerine if your skin is on the oily side.

2 tbsp dried or 4 tbsp fresh chopped nettle, fennel, peppermint, or rosemary

1¼ cups/275 ml boiling water

⅓ cup/90 ml vodka

2 tbsp/30 ml glycerine (for dry or normal skin)

4 drops essential oil (optional)

1 Place the herb in a pitcher or bowl and pour on the boiling water. Cover and leave until cold.
2 Strain into a sterilized bottle. Add the vodka, glycerine, and oil. Shake well.
3 Store in a refrigerator, and shake well before use. Use within one month.

CITRUS BODY TONER Ⓐ

RECIPE

Cold citrus extract will freshen the body after a bath or shower, and close the pores. Omit the glycerine if your skin is on the oily side.

2 lemons

2 oranges

2½ cups/575 ml water

⅔ cup/150 ml vodka

2 tbsp/30 ml glycerine (for dry or normal skin)

1 Finely chop the lemons and oranges into pieces, and place in a saucepan with the water. Bring to the boil, cover and simmer for 15 minutes. Cool and strain.

2 Transfer the liquid to a sterilized bottle. Add the vodka and glycerine, and shake well. Store in a refrigerator. Use within a month. Shake before use.

HERBAL MILK BODY CONDITIONER Ⓝ Ⓞ

RECIPE

This lotion will make your skin feel soft and smooth. The lemon corrects the acid balance. Use it as both toner and moisturizer.

2½ cups/575 ml milk

2 tbsp dried elderflowers, linden, or chamomile flowers

juice 1 lemon

1 Place the milk and flowers in a saucepan and bring gently to a boil.

2 Remove the pan from the heat and let the milk get quite cold.

3 Strain the milk into a bowl and add the lemon juice. Use immediately.

4 Stand in a bath or shower, and sponge the milk over your body. Leave for 15 minutes.

COCOA BUTTER AND CHAMOMILE BODY CREAM Ⓝ Ⓞ

RECIPE

For extra perfume, add several drops of essential oil at the same time as the vitamin E capsule.

1 tbsp dried chamomile flowers

⅔ cup/150 ml boiling water

2 tbsp/30 ml cocoa butter

2 tbsp/30 ml lanolin

one 250 iu vitamin E capsule

⅓ cup/90 ml almond or sunflower oil

1 Place the chamomile flowers in a pitcher or bowl and pour on the boiling water. Cover and leave until cold. Strain.

2 Place the cocoa butter and lanolin in the top of a double boiler or into a bowl set in a saucepan of water. Melt them gently together on a low heat.

3 Prick the vitamin E capsule and squeeze it into the cocoa butter and lanolin.

4 Gradually beat in the oil, then 4 tbsp/60 ml of the chamomile infusion.

5 Beat with an electric beater until the lotion is cold.

6 Transfer the cream to a sterilized pot or jar and cover. Use within three months.

HONEY AND MARIGOLD BODY LOTION Ⓝ Ⓞ

RECIPE

The soothing and healing qualities of marigolds are combined with lanolin, honey, and oils in this fragrant lotion.

2 tbsp dried marigold flowers

⅔ cup/150 ml boiling water

2 tbsp/30 ml lanolin

2 tbsp/30 ml coconut oil

2 tsp/10 ml honey

⅓ cup/90 ml olive or sunflower oil

1 Place half the marigold flowers in a pitcher or bowl and pour on the boiling water. Cover and leave until cold. Strain.

2 Place the rest of the marigold flowers into the top of a double boiler or into a bowl set in a saucepan of water. Add the lanolin and coconut oil. Melt them gently together on a low heat.

3 Beat in the honey, then the oil and 4 tbsp/60 ml of the marigold infusion.

4 Remove entirely from the heat and beat with an electric beater until cold.

5 Transfer the lotion to a sterilized pot or jar and cover. Use within two months.

CARMELITE WATER Ⓐ

This is more expensive to make than Hungary water as the vodka is not diluted. Use it sparingly as a body splash or cologne. Angelica is a herb that is quite hard to find unless you grow it yourself. There is no alternative to angelica

1¼ cups/275 ml vodka

3 tbsp dried or 6 tbsp fresh chopped angelica leaves and stalks

3 tbsp dried or 6 tbsp fresh chopped lemon balm leaves

1 tbsp coriander seeds, bruised

1 nutmeg, cut into chips

2 tbsp cloves

4 x 1 inch/2.5 cm pieces cinnamon stick

1 Pour the vodka into a jar.
2 Add the remaining ingredients, cover tightly and shake.
3 Leave in a warm place for three weeks, shaking every day.
4 Strain into a sterilized bottle and store in a cool place. Use within six months.

CARMELITE WATER

Carmelite water was invented in 1611 by Carmelite monks in Paris who called it Eau de Carmes. In the seventeenth century, lemon balm was a fashionable ingredient in many perfumes made for the wealthy, and the monks made use of their distilling skills to make money for their order. Carmelite water was used as a perfume and toilet water, and was also taken internally as a cordial. Louis XVI was the last King of France to grant the monks a patent for the water's manufacture. Since then, a number of recipes have been published.

Elbows

Sticking out at your sides, elbows can easily be left out of beauty treatments. Sometimes they develop a hard skin that needs tending to. Rub them frequently with a cut lemon, or oatmeal or ground almonds moistened with plain yogurt. Massaging them with one of the following can also help: equal parts glycerine and rosewater; a combination of 1 tbsp/15 ml each olive oil and lemon juice, plus 1 tsp/5 ml honey; sea salt moistened with a little oil. Try the "Elbow softener" on page 89.

TONING AND MOISTURIZING

The simplest way to tone your skin and close the pores after a bath or shower is to splash yourself with cold water. However, for something a little more special, try one of the refreshing fruit- or alcohol-based toners from pages 91-92.

Try to apply a moisturizer after every bath or shower. If you don't have the time, moisturize your body at least once a week.

In the winter, it is especially easy to neglect those areas that are hidden beneath layers of clothes. If you don't use a moisturizer, you may find dry, flaky patches appearing.

THE EFFECTS OF THE SUN

A certain amount of sunshine is essential for good health because it is a rich source of vitamin D. However, the sun's rays can also be harmful, so soak them up in moderation and always protect your skin.

Sunlight contains three types of ultraviolet rays: ultraviolet A, B, and C. When they come into contact with your skin they stimulate the epidermis to produce a shield called melanin. This is the brown pigment that produces a tan. The fairer the skin, the less melanin is produced, and so fair-skinned people are at a greater risk of sunburn than those with dark skin. Black and Asian skins are protected by a constant supply of melanin, but they can still burn and so should be protected.

Another of the body's defenses is for the epidermis to thicken. If this happens frequently your skin can lose some of its elasticity and show early signs of aging such as forming wrinkles or becoming very dry. In fact, the sun is probably responsible for 90 percent of the aging effects suffered by your skin.

Skin burns as a result of ultraviolet B rays hitting the surface and literally cooking it. Even though the burn may eventually turn brown it is not technically a suntan, since it is formed by a different method. Severe sunburn can cause skin cancer later in life. This is because the ultraviolet damage may cause the cells the

body makes to repair the burned ones to mutate and form as cancer cells.

The sun's rays are at their most damaging during the summer, in the middle of the day, in high altitudes, and in hot climates. However, ultraviolet rays are always there so always protect your exposed skin.

Diet

The production of melanin uses up your body's supplies of vitamin B, so eat plenty of things that contain it such as whole grain bread, other unrefined carbohydrates, avocado, dark-green vegetables, eggs, lean meat, and brewer's yeast. A healthy skin also needs a good supply of vitamin C, so eat fresh fruits and salads every day. Drink plenty of water, both in the sun and after, to prevent your system from dehydrating.

Protection

A few years back, the Australians developed the catch phrase "slip, slap, slop," meaning slip on a T-shirt, slap on a hat and slop on the sun screen. It is something that we should all adopt. When the sun is at its hottest, either stay indoors or cover up as much as possible. A wide-brimmed hat will protect the face, hair, and the back of the neck.

Quick Fixes

• Make up 1 quart/1 liter strong herbal decoction or infusion and add it to the bath water after you have run the bath. About 1¼ cups/275 ml milk can be substituted for the same quantity of water.

• To soothe mild sunburn, gently spread one of the following over the affected area, leave for 15 minutes, then rinse off with lukewarm water: mashed or blended cucumber; crushed strawberries; plain yogurt; grated raw potato; cotton balls soaked in strong tea or cold tea bags; 1 egg white beaten with 1 tsp/5 ml each witch hazel and honey; equal parts sesame or olive oil and vinegar.

If you want to tan sensibly, do not overdo it on the first day. Choose your time in the sun with care: either early morning or late afternoon and stay out for only about 15 minutes. Gradually build up your exposure time after that. The rest of the time, find some shade and stay there.

Always use a sun screen with a sun protection factor (SPF) that matches your skin. The SPF number is designed to give you an indication of the length of time you can stay out in the sun without burning. The average person can stay in the sun safely for just ten minutes without protection. To work out the length of time you can stay out in the sun, multiply the SPF number by ten. So, a sunblock with an SPF of 15 should allow you to stay in the sun safely for 150 minutes (two and a half hours). However, it is not quite that simple because everyone is different, and some skins can withstand far more sun than others. Use the SPF as a rough guide.

When in doubt, buy a block with a high SPF and gradually reduce it if you find your skin is tolerant of the sun and is not burned or irritated.

Aftersun

When you come in from the sun, have a cool bath or shower to refresh your skin and lower its temperature. Then splash on an all-over skin toner and moisturize well. If you are burned, there is nothing you can do that will significantly speed up the healing process, but there are things that might help you feel better.

Skin lighteners

Once a tan fades, it can leave your skin looking sallow and tired. To lighten and freshen your complexion, use an exfoliant, or one of the following skin lighteners. Freckles can also be lightened by regular use of herbal face washes and toners. (Freckles should not be regarded as a problem, but some people would do anything to get rid of them.) Lightening herbs include chamomile, elderflower, and parsley You can also try applying crushed strawberries or grapes to your face for 15 minutes, before washing them off with lukewarm water.

RICH AFTERSUN CREAM WITH ELDERFLOWER Ⓐ

Elderflowers and lavender oil will soothe skin that has been exposed to the sun. This soft, rich cream can be rubbed all over the body.

2 tsp dried elderflowers

⅔ cup/150 ml water

2 tbsp/30 ml cocoa butter

2 tbsp/30 ml beeswax

½ cup/125 ml sesame or safflower oil

6 drops lavender oil

1 Place the elderflowers and water in a saucepan and bring to a boil. Cover and simmer for five minutes. Leave to cool, then strain off the decoction.
2 Place the cocoa butter and beeswax in the top of a double boiler or into a bowl set in a saucepan of water. Melt them gently on a low heat.
3 Gradually beat in the sesame or safflower oil.
4 Remove entirely from the heat and beat in 2 tbsp/30 ml of the elderflower decoction.
5 Beat in the lavender oil. Leave to cool, stirring frequently.
6 Transfer the cream to a sterilized pot or jar. Cover when completely cold, and use within one month.

AFTERSUN OIL WITH TEA Ⓐ

Tea cools the skin and helps to maintain a tan. The sesame oil enriches the skin to prevent it from drying.

4 tbsp/60 ml sesame oil

4 tbsp/60 ml coconut oil

4 tbsp/60 ml strong plain tea

4 drops lavender oil

1 Place the sesame and coconut oils in the top of a double boiler or into a bowl set in a saucepan of water. Melt them together.
2 Beat in the tea.
3 Remove entirely from the heat and beat in the lavender oil.
4 Transfer the mixture to a sterilized bottle and shake well before use.

CUCUMBER COOLER Ⓐ

Keep this cooling lotion in the refrigerator so it is always ready to splash on your skin after days in the sun.

1 cucumber

2 tbsp/30 ml glycerine

2 tbsp/30 ml rosewater

1 Finely chop the cucumber by hand, or in a blender or food processor.
2 Strain off the juice and add the glycerine and rosewater.
3 Transfer the lotion to a sterilized bottle and shake well.
4 Store in a refrigerator and use within one week. Shake well before use.

COOLING BATH BAG Ⓐ

For this recipe you will need to make a muslin, cheesecloth, or cotton bag. Follow the instuctions for "Herbal bath bags" on page 85.

4 tbsp fine oatmeal

4 tbsp dried or 2 heads fresh elderflowers

⅔ cup/150 ml cider vinegar

1 Fill a bag with the oatmeal and elderflower mixture.
2 Run a lukewarm bath, placing the bag of oatmeal under the running water.
3 Add the cider vinegar to the filled bath, and swish it around in the water.
4 While you are soaking, gently squeeze the bag of oatmeal to make the bath water soft and milky.

OATMEAL POULTICE FOR SUNBURN Ⓐ

This poultice will soothe skin that has had too much sun. If you don't have muslin, use a piece of thin cotton or old handkerchiefs instead.

2 tbsp fine oatmeal

4 tbsp/60 ml plain yogurt

1 tbsp/15 ml witch hazel

1 tbsp/15 ml lemon juice

1 Place the oatmeal in a bowl and mix in the yogurt, witch hazel, and lemon juice.
2 Spread the treatment over a piece of muslin, cover it with another piece of muslin, and lay it on your skin. Leave for 30 minutes.
3 Remove the poultice and wipe your skin with a cotton ball soaked in milk or buttermilk. Leave to dry.

FACE LIGHTENER Ⓝ Ⓞ

Use this to lighten freckles or freshen a fading suntan.

2 tbsp/30 ml plain yogurt

1 tsp/5 ml lemon juice

1 tsp/5 ml preserved grated horseradish

1 Combine all the ingredients and spread the mixture over your face. Leave for 15 minutes.
2 Rinse off with warm water, then splash your face with cold water or an herbal toner (see page 91).
3 The treatment is very drying so use an oil-rich moisturizer such as "Vitamin-enriched moisturizer" or "Cocoa butter moisturizer" (see page 39) after the treatment, or massage your face with pure almond, sesame, or olive oil.

SKIN-LIGHTENING FACE MASK Ⓞ

This mask is very tautening, and so is excellent for oily skin. If you have a dry or normal skin, make sure that you use a rich moisturizer afterwards.

1 egg white

juice ½ lemon

1 Place the egg white and lemon juice in the top of a double boiler or in a bowl set in a saucepan of water over a low heat. Stir together until the mixture thickens. Remove entirely from the heat and leave until cold.
2 Spread the mixture over your face and leave for as long as possible—two hours would be ideal.
3 Rinse off the mixture with tepid water. Splash the face with cold water, pat dry, tone, and moisturize.

SESAME OIL

Sesame oil is produced from the small, oil-rich seeds of the sesame plant (*Sesamum indicum*). The best quality oil is extracted by a process called cold pressing. This consists of pressing the seeds with a hydraulic press without applying additional heat. The extracted oil is then filtered with a screen to remove coarse matter.

Cold-pressed sesame oil is the best to use for all skin treatments. It also has the ability to filter out some of the sun's harmful rays, but not enough to prevent burning. It is best reserved for aftersun treatments.

With a good-quality base oil, and a selection of natural essential oils, you can create perfumes to suit your personality and your moods.

ESSENTIAL OILS

Essential oils are extracted by distillation or by expression (pressing). Oils can be extracted from all parts of a plant: flowers, buds, leaves and stems, barks, woods, roots, seeds, and resins. Essential oils are now widely available and can be bought from herbalists, drugstores, health food stores and aromatherapy suppliers. Keep essential oils in a cool, dark place and use them within two years.

The effectiveness of plant oils has been known for centuries, but it is only relatively recently that this knowledge has been backed up by scientific evidence. Essential oils have been found to be antiseptic, antibiotic, anti-inflammatory, and antiviral and their use stimulates the body's immune system. They can also have effects on mood and general attitude. As a result, your home-produced perfumes can be scented and therapeutic.

Besides natural plant oils, there are also synthetic oils, sometimes called nature-identical oils. Nature-

You will soon come to recognize oils, and discover which scents you like best. Here are some combinations to try:

• Sweet and exotic with a hint of citrus: 8 drops jasmine, 6 drops lemon, 4 drops patchouli.
• Fresh and sweet: 4 drops neroli, 4 drops lavender, 2 drops spearmint.
• Oriental with a hint of lemon: 4 drops sandalwood, 3 drops lemon verbena, 4 drops musk, 2 drops frankincense.
• Floral with a hint of spice: 6 drops jasmine, 3 drops orange, 2 drops sandalwood.
• Rich and sweet: 8 drops rose, 4 drops jasmine, 2 drops bergamot.

• Sweet and floral: 6 drops ylang-ylang, 3 drops clary sage, 2 drops lemon, 2 drops lavender.
• Woody and sensual: 8 drops musk, 4 drops sandalwood, 3 drops oakmoss, 2 drops patchouli.
• Fresh and citrusy: 3 drops grapefruit, 3 drops lemon, 2 drops spearmint, 1 drop bergamot.

What you will need:
small dark glass bottle
1 tsp/5 ml or 2 tsp/10 ml measuring
   spoon
small funnel
several droppers
strips of blotting paper
2 tsp/10 ml jojoba oil
selection of essential oils

1 Choose three or four essential oils. Decide which are the top, middle, and base notes, and which you would like to be the most dominant.
2 Place drops of the oils, in the proportion in which you would like to use them, onto a strip of blotting paper. Leave for five minutes, then sniff to see if you have achieved the desired effect. Correct if necessary.
3 Pour the jojoba oil into the bottle. Add up to 20 drops essential oil in the proportions that you have worked out. Cover. Shake well. Sniff to test. Correct, if necessary, adding only one extra drop of oil at a time.
4 Leave the perfume for 12 hours in a cool, dark place for the blend to mature. Use within two months.

identical oils include certain rose oils and neroli oil, which are made synthetically because the pure equivalents are so expensive, and musk oil which, if naturally produced, would have to be of animal origin.

Do remember that if an oil seems expensive, a few drops, once mixed with a carrier oil, will go a long way.

Important Before creating a perfume, test for sensitivity by placing one drop of each of the chosen oils on your arm. Leave for an hour, and if they cause an allergic reaction do not use.

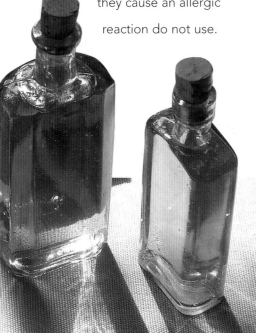

SCENTS AND BLENDING

The scents of essential oils can be divided into types or families. These are floral, chypre (woody and earthy), green (fresh and clean), and oriental.

In the nineteenth century a Frenchman named Piesse decided that scents for perfumery could be classified in a scale similar to a musical scale. His fairly complicated system has since been simplified and, today, perfume scents are divided into top, middle and base notes. A well-blended perfume must contain all three, and the final effect depends on the balance between them.

Top notes are fresh and light. They are the first scents that you detect in a blended perfume, and are often the most volatile.

Middle notes usually form the main character of the blend. They have a lasting scent that becomes apparent after that of the top notes. This is then complemented by the base notes.

Base notes are rich and heavy, they are the last to be detected and probably the longest to linger. They also have fixative qualities and prevent the lighter scents from dissipating too quickly.

THE PIESSE SCALE

Scent	Type	Note	Scent	Type	Note
Bergamot	green	top	Mandarin	green	top
Carnation	floral	middle	Marjoram	green	middle
Cedarwood	chypre	middle	Musk	chypre	base
Clary sage	green	middle	Neroli	floral	base
Cypress	chypre	middle	Oakmoss	chypre	base
Frankincense	oriental	base	Patchouli	oriental	base
Geranium	floral/green	middle	Peppermint	green	top
Jasmine	floral	base	Rose	floral	base
Lavender	green	middle	Rosemary	green	middle
Lemon	green	top	Sandalwood	oriental	base
Lemon balm	green	middle	Spearmint	green	top
Lemon verbena	green	middle	Vanilla	chypre	base
Lime	green	top	Ylang-ylang	combination	base

H A N D S

cleanse

exfoliate

massage

manicure

exercise

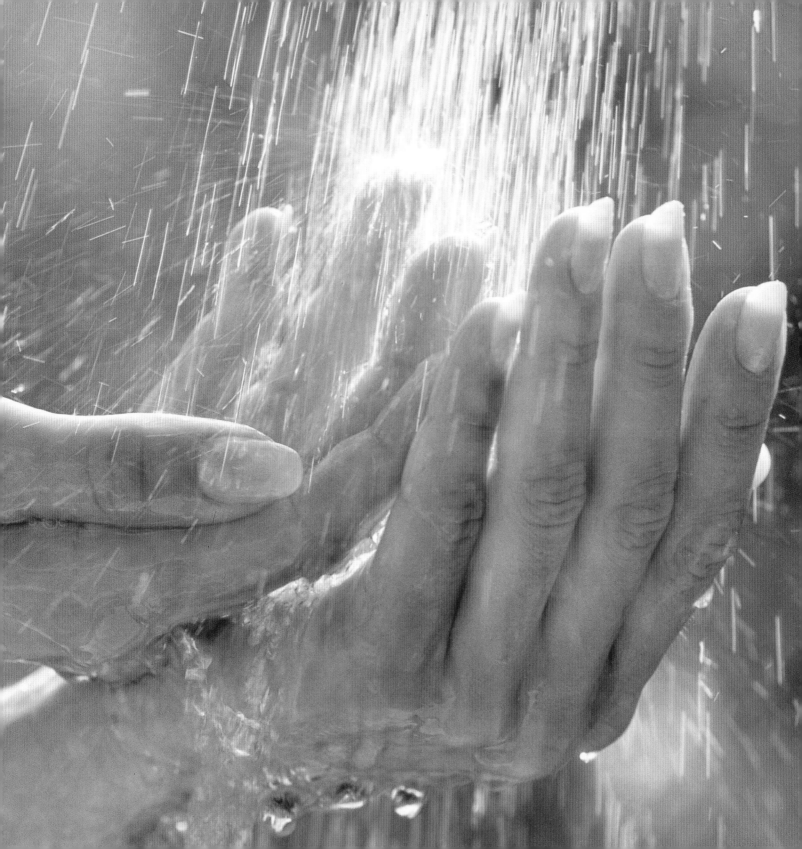

Hands are constantly exposed to extremes of the weather, and are prey to a variety of enemies, so always try to protect them. Wear warm gloves in cold weather to prevent chapping; in the summer, use a sun screen on your hands, especially if you are often outside.

Doing gardening and other jobs outdoors can lead to scratched or chapped hands. The best solution is to wear gardening gloves or heavier industrial ones, depending on the job. Where you find it impossible to use gloves, such as when pricking out seedlings that need delicate handling, use a barrier cream to protect your hands from the worst of the dirt. You will find a recipe for this in the following pages.

Indoors, wear rubber gloves for washing the dishes, handwashing clothes, and when cleaning around the house—especially if using chemical cleaners. If you keep your hands in water for long periods, or if your hands are constantly in and out of water, the skin can become wrinkly, and the nails swollen.

Chlorine can dry out your hands and nails so, after you have been swimming, dry your hands well and use a rich moisture cream.

CLEANSING AND EXFOLIATING

Use gentle soaps on your hands, even after dirty work. Instead of alkaline-based soaps choose those enriched with oils or glycerine. Other efficient hand cleansers include oatmeal, cornmeal, bran, or ground almonds. Keep one of these, either alone or combined, (for example almonds and oatmeal), in a small pot and moisten it with a little water to use.

To keep the backs of your hands soft and smooth, exfoliate them regularly. Apply one of the following simple exfoliants by massaging it into the back of each hand with small, circular movements for about one minute: 4 tbsp/60 ml sunflower or almond oil mixed with 1 tbsp sea salt; oatmeal, cornmeal, or ground almonds

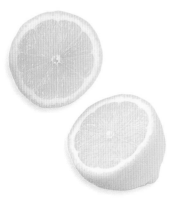

moistened with plain yogurt and a little cider vinegar or lemon juice; white sugar moistened with hot water. Rinse off with warm water, and apply a rich lotion or moisturizing cream

NAILS

Your nails are are made of a hard material that is almost pure protein. If they are thin, dry or brittle it is usually the result of your health rather than external treatment, so take care of your diet. Eat an adequate amount of protein, nuts, and foods that contain vitamin A. It is also a good idea to drink 1 tsp/5 ml each brewer's yeast and honey in a cup of hot water daily.

All the advice that applies to your hands applies to your nails, too. If you are not going

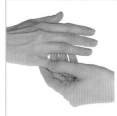
to wear gloves for dirty work such as gardening, push barrier cream under your nails, or scratch on a piece of cocoa butter or a bar of soap. This will help prevent grit from getting under the nails. If your nails are still dirty when you return indoors, dig them into the soap before washing your hands. Use a nailbrush, preferably one with a single layer of bristles on the back, to get rid of the remaining dirt.

Nail polish tends to dry out your nails, so don't leave it on too long and always use an oil-based remover. False nails and their glue can damage your own nails underneath. It is better to look after the real ones.

BARRIER CREAM Ⓐ

Rub this onto your hands before tackling tough jobs in the house or around the garden.

1 egg yolk

2 tbsp/30 ml sunflower oil

fuller's earth or kaolin powder

1 pair old cotton gloves (optional)

1 Place the egg yolk in a bowl and beat in the oil.
2 Gradually mix in enough fuller's earth or kaolin powder to make a smooth paste. Use immediately. (Gloves will help keep the cream on your hands.)

OIL AND LEMON STAIN REMOVER Ⓐ

This is a simple but effective method of removing stubborn stains from your hands.

1 tbsp/15 ml sunflower oil

1 tbsp/15 ml lemon juice

1 tsp white sugar

1 Beat the ingredients together.
2 Massage into the stains on your hands.
3 Rinse off with tepid water. Pat dry, then apply hand lotion or cream.

GROUND ALMOND HAND TREATMENT Ⓐ

Once a month, treat yourself to a treatment that will exfoliate and soften your hands.

3 tbsp ground almonds

1 egg yolk

2 tbsp/30 ml olive oil

1 tbsp/15 ml rosewater

1 pair generously fitting old cotton gloves

1 pair plastic gloves (optional)

1 Place the almonds in a bowl.
2 Beat in the egg yolk, then the oil and rosewater.
3 Massage the mixture into your hands.
4 Put on the cotton gloves and leave the mixture as long as possible. Overnight is best. If you are doing this during the daytime, wear plastic gloves over the top to prevent the cream from oozing through.

MARIGOLD HAND CREAM Ⓐ

This is a beautiful yellow color and gently fragrant.

¾ cup/175 ml petroleum jelly

1 tbsp/15 ml beeswax

1 tbsp/15 ml lanolin

2 tbsp dried or 4 tbsp fresh marigold flowers

1 Place the petroleum jelly, beeswax, and lanolin in a small casserole and melt on a low heat.
2 Add the marigold flowers.
3 Cover the casserole and place in a preheated oven at 200°F/100°C for three hours.
4 Strain through muslin or a nylon sieve directly into a sterilized pot or jar. Cover when completely cold and use within three months.

ROSEWATER HAND SOFTENER Ⓐ

Use this non-greasy preparation like hand cream.

2 tbsp corn flour

½ cup/125 ml rosewater

2 tbsp/30 ml glycerine

juice ½ lemon

1 In a bowl, mix the corn flour with 4 tbsp/60 ml of the rosewater.
2 Pour the remaining rosewater into a saucepan with the glycerine. Heat gently.
3 Stir in the corn flour mixture and the lemon juice. Simmer, stirring, until the mixture is thick. Remove the pan from the heat.
4 Transfer the mixture to a sterilized pot or jar. Cover when completely cold. Store in a refrigerator and use within two weeks.

CUCUMBER AND GLYCERINE HAND LOTION Ⓐ

Like all glycerine hand lotions, this one isn't greasy. The cucumber makes it very moisturizing.

1 inch/2.5 cm piece cucumber

2 tbsp/30 ml glycerine

2 tbsp/30 ml rosewater

2 tbsp/30 ml vodka or brandy

1 Peel, finely chop, and mash the cucumber in a bowl.
2 Add the remaining ingredients to the cucumber pulp.
3 Transfer to a sterilized pot or jar and store in a refrigerator. Use within one week.

CONDITIONING MASSAGE CREAM Ⓐ

Use this massage cream once a week to keep your hands soft and smooth. The almonds and oatmeal slough off dead skin cells, and the herbal infusion is soothing. If you don't have ground almonds, add an extra teaspoon of oatmeal.

1 tsp dried lady's mantle, elderflowers, or marigolds

⅓ cup/90 ml boiling water

1 tbsp fine oatmeal

1 tsp ground almonds

1 tsp/5 ml almond, avocado, or olive oil

1 tsp/5 ml glycerine

1 tsp/5 ml lemon juice

1 Place the herb into a sterilized pitcher or bowl. Pour on the boiling water, cover and leave until cold. Strain.
2 Place the oatmeal and ground almonds in a bowl and mix in the oil, glycerine, lemon juice, and 1 tbsp/15 ml of the herbal infusion. Use immediately.
3 Massage the mixture into your hands. After massaging, leave the mixture on for 20 minutes.
4 Rinse off with tepid water and apply a hand cream if wished.

LEMON AND LADY'S MANTLE HAND LOTION Ⓝ Ⓞ

This a light, non-greasy lotion both softens and whitens the hands. Lavender, marigold flowers, or elderflowers can be used instead of the lady's mantle to make the herbal decoction. Alternatively, use rosewater.

1 tsp dried or 1 tbsp fresh chopped lady's mantle

⅔ cup/150 ml water

4 tbsp/60 ml lemon juice

4 tbsp/60 ml glycerine

2 tbsp/30 ml vodka

1 Place the lady's mantle and water in a saucepan and bring to a boil. Simmer for five minutes. Cool and strain.
2 Pour 4 tbsp/60 ml of the decoction into a sterilized bottle. Add the other ingredients and shake well. Store in a refrigerator and use within one week.
3 Apply daily to your hands, massaging it in well. Shake before use.

LADY'S MANTLE (*Alchemilla vulgaris*)

Lady's mantle is a herb that has been used mainly for menstrual disorders, but which also has soothing and wound-healing properties. It is an attractive herb with large, circular leaves, rather like fans, and branches of small yellow flowers. In the herb garden it grows to the height of about 20 inches/50 cm, and likes a moist soil.

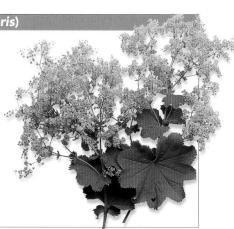

TREATMENT FOR CHAPPED HANDS Ⓐ

Warm milk is a soothing treatment for chapped hands. Make up a simple, rich cream to use afterwards.

For the cream:

3 tbsp/45 ml lanolin

1 tbsp/15 ml olive oil

one 250 iu vitamin E capsule (optional)

For the treatment:

1¼ cups/275 ml whole milk

2 hand-sized pieces cotton wool

1 Place the lanolin and olive oil in the top of a double boiler or into a bowl set in a saucepan of water. Melt them together on a low heat, stirring frequently.
2 Prick the vitamin E capsule and squeeze the contents into the saucepan.
3 Remove the cream from the heat and cool it, beating frequently.
4 Transfer the cream to a sterilized pot or jar. Cover when completely cold and use within one month.
5 Pour the warmed milk into a bowl. Soak the cotton wool pieces in the milk. Lay one on each hand. Keep them there for 20 minutes. Massage any wetness left on your hands into the skin.
6 Massage in some of the cream.

NAIL-CONDITIONING MASSAGE CREAM

Massage this into your nails every day for a week, and they will become healthy and strong. After that, use once a week to maintain the effect.

1 egg yolk

2 tbsp/30 ml almond, avocado, or olive oil

1 tsp/5 ml honey

¼ tsp sea salt

1 Place the egg yolk in a bowl and beat in the oil, honey, and salt.
2 Use immediately, massaging the mixture into your nails, taking about five minutes for each hand. Do not wash off the residue until the following morning.

NAIL-STRENGTHENING CREAM

Horsetail is a renowned nail strengthener. Massage this cream into your fingernails daily.

1 tbsp dried or 2 tbsp fresh chopped horsetail

4 tbsp/60 ml boiling water

1 tbsp/15 ml cocoa butter

1 tbsp/15 ml lanolin

1 Place the horsetail in a bowl and pour on the boiling water. Cover and leave until cold. Strain.
2 Place the cocoa butter and lanolin in the top of a double boiler or into a bowl set in a saucepan of water. Melt them gently together on a low heat.
3 Beat in 1 tbsp/15 ml of the horsetail infusion.
4 Remove entirely from the heat and beat until the cream has cooled.
5 Transfer the cream to a sterilized pot. Cover when completely cold and use within two months.

HORSETAIL (*Equisetum arvense*)

Horsetail is a spectacular plant that in appearance lives up to its folk name of bottlebrush. It is tall, with very thin, spiky leaves, that make it look like a brush or feather duster. In prehistoric times, it grew as tall as a tree, but today it can be found up to 3 feet/1 meter high. Horsetail is rich in silica, making it an excellent external treatment for broken or weak nails.

Horsetail is toxic in large doses, and should never be taken internally.

MANICURE

Manicured nails greatly enhance the look of your hands. Try to find time once a week for a treatment.

What you will need:

cotton balls

emery board

⅔ cup/150 ml warm water or infusion of horsetail

bowl

4 tbsp/60 ml sunflower, olive, or almond oil

cotton swabs, or orange sticks wrapped in cotton

towel

nail buffer, soft cloth, or piece of chamois leather

hand cream or lotion

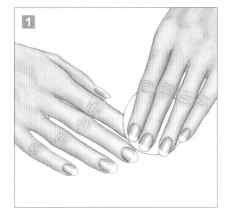

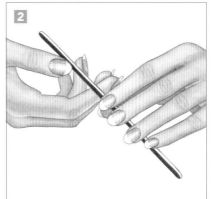

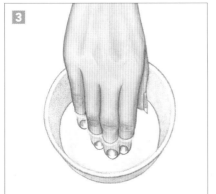

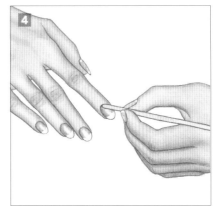

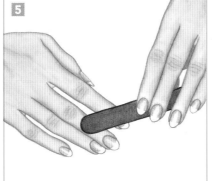

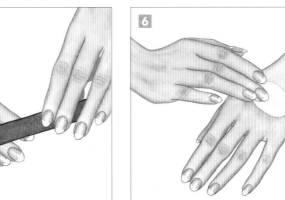

1 Remove any nail polish.
2 Shape the nails with an emery board, not a metal nail file. Work in one direction only and do not take them too far down at the corners. Aim for almond-shaped or squared nails.
3 Pour the warm water or infusion into a bowl. Add the oil. Dabble your fingertips in this for ten minutes. Dry gently.
4 Using a cotton swab or orange stick wrapped in cotton, gently press back the cuticles. (They should never be cut.)
5 Buff your nails.
6 Massage in hand cream or lotion.

FEET

soothe

invigorate

moisturize

exercise

massage

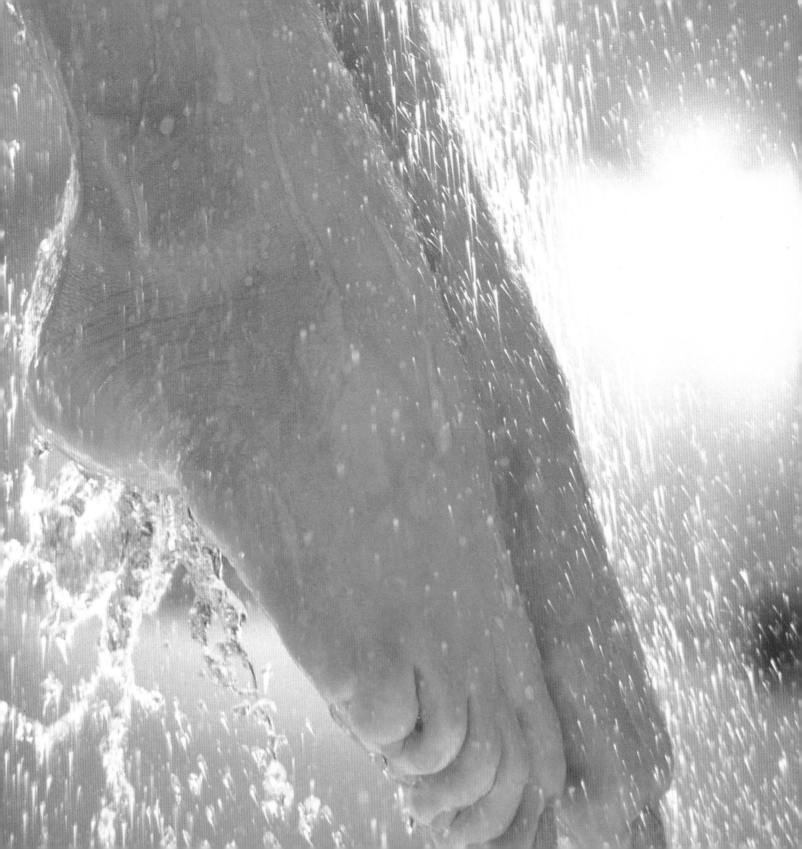

Your feet and legs support you throughout the day, helping you to walk, run, climb, and dance, so give them some attention. Feet have to take the weight of your whole body and, in order to do this efficiently, they need to spread out naturally. It pays, therefore, to buy well-fitting shoes that give you a certain amount of support. If you have normal or narrow feet, this will be relatively easy. If you have wide feet, you may have to look further.

We humans were not designed to walk on our toes: high heels make us lean forward and stick out our buttocks at an awkward angle. By all means wear high heels for special occasions and when you want to feel elegant, but choose something flatter for every day.

Encasing your feet in stretchy hose or stockings also constricts the toes, so kick off your shoes, take off the nylons, and walk barefoot whenever you can. Wriggle your toes occasionally to keep them supple.

Activities that help to keep legs and feet in shape include swimming, cycling, walking, yoga, or stretching exercises

Legs have fewer sebaceous glands than any other part of the body, and the calves are often the place where uncared-for skin begins to look dry and flaky. So, whenever you moisturize your body, pay particular attention to your legs, especially if you have been out in the sun.

Exfoliate your legs with the "Salt and oil body rub" (see page 89) or by rubbing with a pumice stone, loofah, or hand mitt when you are in the bath. If your knees look dry and flaky, use the "Elbow softener" treatment given on page 89.

Foot baths

If you feel brave and are in need of a good body toner or early morning reviver, try a cold foot bath. Stand in the bath and run the cold tap until the water comes up to your ankles and, if you can stand it, up to your calves. Then

Quick Fixes

• Here's a simple booster for tired legs and feet: lie down with your feet above your head for ten minutes then, with a light coating of oil on your hands, gently massage each leg in turn with continual movements from ankle to knee.

quickly towel yourself dry. You can also hold the shower nozzle and sit with just your feet in the shower stream.

Herbal foot baths revive and relieve aching feet, and make the rest of the body feel good, too. The skin on your feet is surprisingly absorbent. To try this out, rub a small amount of peppermint oil on your soles. Within about 20 minutes you will begin to taste peppermint. With this in mind, add herbs to your foot bath that suit your needs. For a list, see "Herbs to add to your bath" on pages 78-79. Dried herbs should be tied in a piece of muslin or cotton. Fresh herbs can be used on the sprig. This will prevent too much mess. For the method, see the recipes below.

After any kind of bath, always dry your feet well, especially between the toes, to prevent infections such as athlete's foot.

SOLVING PROBLEMS

Corns form as a protection against tight shoes or constant rubbing, so in addition to treating the corn try to sort out the cause. Small corns can usually be dealt with by using a pumice stone when you use a foot bath or have a bath. You can also try the garlic treatment. Rub the corn with a cut clove of garlic, then take one sliver of garlic and secure it onto the corn with plaster or a bandage. Replace it daily until the corn disappears. If this doesn't work, consult a chiropodist.

If you suffer from smelly feet, take a daily foot bath made with deodorizing herbs such as basil or lovage, and dry and powder your feet well afterwards.

FOOT MASSAGE

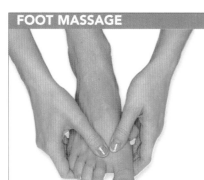

Use a base oil such as almond, avocado, jojoba, or wheat germ. Choose either refreshing or relaxing essential oils to add to it.

What you will need:
towel
base oil

Method:

1 Rest your feet on a towel. Coat your hands and feet in a thin film of oil.

2 Place both hands either side of one foot, with your thumbs on top and all fingers underneath. Place your thumbs in the center of your foot and gradually draw them outwards to the sides of the foot. Do this six times.

3 With your hands in the same position, massage the tops of your foot with small circular movements of your thumbs.

4 Turn your foot over and rest it on your other leg. Place your hands in the same position, but this time with your thumbs on the soles of your feet. Massage with the same circular movements.

5 Press your thumbs firmly all over the sole of your foot.

6 Hold each toe in turn with your thumb in front and your forefinger underneath. Gently squeeze the toe and give it a firm tug.

7 With your foot upright, hold it with a hand on either side. Stroke with long, slow movements from toe to ankle.

RECIPE REFRESHING HERBAL FOOT BATH

This will relax and refresh tired feet and legs.

1 tsp dried or 1 tbsp fresh rosemary

1 tsp dried or 1 tbsp fresh peppermint

2 tbsp sea salt

enough boiling water to fill bowl

juice ½ lemon

1 Place the herbs in the bowl and add the sea salt.
2 Pour enough boiling water into the bowl to cover your feet.
3 Lay a large towel over the bowl and leave until the water has cooled down sufficiently for you to put your feet into it.
4 Add the lemon juice.
5 Soak your feet in the foot bath for as long as you wish, but don't let the water get cold.

RECIPE HERBAL FOOT BATH TO SOOTHE SORE FEET

Use this after a hard day on your feet.

1 tsp dried or 1 tbsp fresh lavender flowers

1 tbsp dried elderflowers or 2 fresh elderflower heads

1 tbsp dried chamomile or 6 fresh chamomile flowers

enough boiling water to fill bowl

1 Place the herbs in the bowl.
2 Pour enough boiling water into the bowl to cover your feet.
3 Lay a large towel over the bowl and leave until the water has cooled down sufficiently for you to put your feet into it.
4 Soak your feet in the foot bath for as long as you wish, but don't let the water get cold.

RECIPE COMFORTING HERBAL FOOT BATH

This is a foot bath to relax both your feet and your spirits.

1 tsp dried or 1 tbsp fresh lavender flowers

1 tsp dried or 1 tbsp fresh comfrey leaves

8 scented geranium leaves, if available

1 tbsp Epsom salts or washing soda

enough boiling water to fill bowl

1 Place the herbs and the other ingredients in the bowl.
2 Pour enough boiling water into the bowl to cover your feet.
3 Lay a large towel over the bowl and leave until the water has cooled down sufficiently for you to put your feet into it.
4 Soak your feet in the foot bath for as long as you wish, but don't let the water get cold.

SCENTED GERANIUM LEAVES

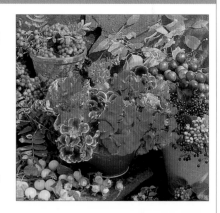

What are often referred to as scented geraniums are in fact pelargoniums, whose beauty is in the shape and fragrance of their leaves. Some are soft and furry, others ridged and deeply cut, and their scents range from fresh mints and lemons to the sweet and resinous.

You can grow scented geraniums in pots, keep them for years, and take cuttings regularly to ensure that you have a good supply of leaves. Keep them indoors in winter and outdoors in summer. Water them regularly, feed in summer and cut them back twice a year to keep them bushy.

Scented geraniums can sometimes be picked up quite cheaply at summer fairs and flea markets. Otherwise, go to a specialist nursery or a herb grower. You need your own supplies as geranium leaves are seldom available dried.

HERBAL FOOT BATH WITH ESSENTIAL OIL

This fragrant foot bath is a treat for the whole body.

hot water

up to 20 drops essential oil of appropriate herbs

2 tbsp sea salt or 1 tbsp Epsom salts (optional)

1 Pour enough hot water into a large bowl to cover your feet.
2 Add essential oils of your choice and swish them about.
3 Add sea salt or Epsom salts, if using.
4 Soak your feet in the foot bath for as long as you wish, but don't let the water get cold.

ROSEMARY AND MARJORAM FOOT OIL

If your feet are aching after walking a long way or dancing all night, give them a massage with this restorative oil.

½ cup/125 ml sunflower oil

4 tbsp/60 ml wheat germ oil

1 tbsp/15 ml cider vinegar

6 drops rosemary oil

6 drops marjoram oil

1 Pour the sunflower and wheat germ oils into a sterilized bottle or jar.
2 Add the cider vinegar and essential oils. Shake well and shake before use.

LAVENDER AND PEPPERMINT FOOT LOTION

After a bath or a foot bath, splash this lotion onto your feet to make them feel cool and fresh.

3 tbsp dried lavender flowers

⅔ cup/150 ml water

5 tbsp/75 ml glycerine

5 tbsp/75 ml vodka

6 drops peppermint oil

1 Place the lavender flowers and water in a saucepan and bring to a boil. Cover and simmer for five minutes. Cool and strain.
2 Pour the decoction into a sterilized bottle or jar and add the glycerine, vodka, and peppermint oil. Shake well and shake before use. Use within two months.

FOOT AND ANKLE EXERCISES

1 Sit on a chair or on the floor. Lift one leg and support it under the knee with your hands.
2 Rotate your foot from the ankle, ten times outwards and ten times inwards. Repeat with the other foot.
3 Hold the first leg up again. Point your toe and hold for a count of five. Bring your toe toward you and push your heel forwards. Hold for five. Repeat three times more. Do the same with the other leg.
4 Shake each lower leg in turn until your foot feels loose.

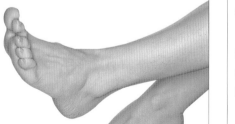

PEPPERMINT (*Mentha piperita*)

The peppermint plant is a variety of mint that has the classic peppermint scent and flavor. It is similar in appearance to ordinary garden mint, the main difference being the red-tinged color of its leaves and stems.

Peppermint is widely grown commercially for its oil and to sell dried as peppermint tea. The relief of fatigue, stress, and muscular pain are some of peppermint's healing properties. It is also highly refreshing. These characteristics make it an ideal addition to foot treatments of all kinds.

TREATMENT FOR ROUGH SKIN

Rough skin on feet is a common problem. Give yourself this treatment several times a week. The cream will keep for two months, so can be made in advance.

For the cream:

2 tbsp/30 ml coconut oil

2 tbsp/30 ml olive oil

1 tbsp/15 ml infusion of marigold, elderflower or nettle, or rosewater

4 drops lavender oil

For the massage:

2 tbsp/30 ml plain yogurt

1 tsp/5 ml cider vinegar

1 To make the cream, pour the oils into the top of a double boiler or into a bowl set in a saucepan of water. Melt them gently together on a low heat.
2 Beat in the infusion or rosewater.
3 Remove entirely from the heat and beat in the lavender oil. Continue to beat until cool.
4 Transfer to a sterilized pot. Cover when completely cold.
5 When you are ready to do the massage, mix the yogurt with the cider vinegar.
6 Massage the mixture into the spots of hard skin on your feet, taking about 15 minutes to do both feet.
7 Rinse off with tepid water. Pat dry and rub in the cream.

CHILBLAIN TREATMENT

Chilblains can are caused by prolonged exposure to cold and damp. Feet and toes become tender, swollen, and itchy. This treatment is rather messy, but effective. After soaking your feet in an infusion of comfrey and marigold, find a place to sit undisturbed for an hour, with a compress of herbs on your feet.

1 tbsp dried comfrey leaves

1 tbsp dried marigold flowers

enough boiling water to fill the bowl

Marigold hand cream (page 104)

1 Tie the comfrey leaves and marigold flowers in a piece of muslin, cheesecloth, or in a large, old handkerchief. Place them in a large bowl. Pour enough boiling water into the bowl to cover your feet. Leave until the water is lukewarm. Squeeze the bag to extract as much from the herbs as possible.
2 Soak your feet in the infusion for ten minutes. Pat them dry. Save the infusion.
3 Sit down and place your feet on an old towel. Unwrap the wet herbs and lay them over the chilblains. Sit there, if possible, for an hour.
4 Remove the herbs and rinse off any excess with the saved infusion. Pat your feet dry.
5 Massage with "Marigold hand cream."

FOOT POWDER

Dust this powder over clean, dry feet to keep them feeling fresh. Make the powder in the bag in which you are going to keep it.

4 oz/125 g unscented baby powder

4 tbsp corn flour

2 tbsp boric acid

6 drops peppermint oil

6 drops tea tree oil

1 Place the baby powder, corn flour, and boric acid in a strong plastic bag.
2 Rub in the peppermint oil and tea tree oil with your fingertips.
3 Store the powder in the bag, and apply with a small dusting puff or cotton balls. Use within two months.

PEDICURE

Feet are neglected far too often. Give them a treat with this simple pedicure.

What you will need:

a prepared foot bath

pumice stone

towel

nail scissors or clippers

emery board

cotton swabs or orange stick with tips wrapped in cotton

almond or sunflower oil

foot powder or lotion

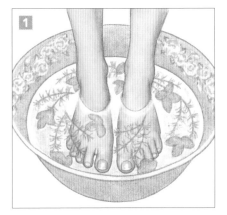

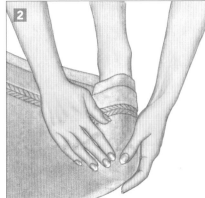

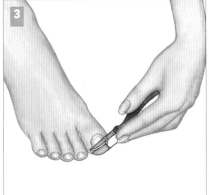

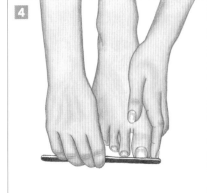

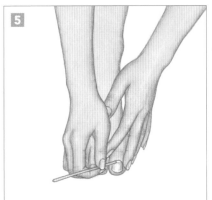

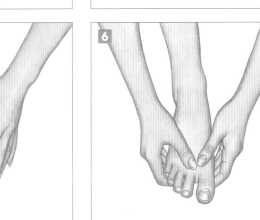

1 Soak your feet for five to ten minutes in an herbal foot bath. While they are soaking, rub any dry skin with a pumice stone.

2 Dry your feet well.

3 Cut your nails with nail scissors or clippers. Do not cut them down at the corners as this causes ingrowing toenails. Make them flat on top or very slightly rounded.

4 Smooth your nails with an emery board, working in one direction.

5 Dip a cotton swab into the oil. Gently press back the cuticles.

6 Massage your feet and dust on foot powder, or coat them in a refreshing foot lotion.

Suppliers

Ingredients for natural beauty preparations are readily available from a variety of sources, such as supermarkets, healthfood stores, herbalists and pharmacists. If you have problems getting hold of an item, contact one of the following companies.

A. C. Moore

609-228-6700

Essential and fragrant oils. Containers. Beeswax. Call for the location of the store nearest you.

Nature's Finest

P.O. Box 10311

Burke, VA 22009-0311

703-978-3925

Large selection of essential and fragrance oils. Catalog. Mail order.

Prima Fleur

1525 E. Francisco Boulevard, Suite 16

San Rafael, CA 94901

415-455-0957

Hard-to-find vegetable oils, natural waxes, hydrosols, herbal-infused oils. Carrier systems such as unscented lotions, creams, and gels. Catalog. Mail order.

Samarkan

936 Peaceportal Drive, Unit 98

Blain, WA 98231-8014

800-260-7401

Cream and milk bases, gels. Phytols and infused oils. Catalog. Mail order.

San Francisco Herb Company

250 14th Street

San Francisco, CA 94103

800-227-4530

Culinary herbs, spices and oils. Organic botanical and fragrant oils. Bags for infusions. Beeswax. Catalog. Mail order.

Tom Thumb Workshops

14100 Lankford Highway

P.O. Box 357

Mappsville, VA 23407

Herbs, spices, essential oils. Catalog. Mail order.

A World of Plenty

P.O. Box 1153

Hermantown, PA 55810-9724

218-729-6761

Essential and fragrance oils, herbs, teas, and tisanes. Catalog. Mail order. Extensive line of organic and wild herbs, extracts, teas, and flower essences. Catalog. Mail order.

Darshan Botanicals

17024 153rd Avenue SE

Yelm, Washington 98597

888-321-4372

Full line of essential oils. Catalog. Mail order.

The Essence of Life

7106 NDCBU

Taos, NM 87571

505-758-7941

Distiller of exotic flowers of India. Full range of essential oils. Mail order.

Kiehl's

103 Third Avenue

New York, NY 10003

212-677-3171

Essential oils. Catalog. Mail order.

Lavender Lane

7337 #1 Roseville Road

Sacramento, CA 95842

916-334-4400

Essential oils, waxes, powders, rosewater. Dried flowers and herbs. Bags to contain infusions. Bottles and jars. Fine quality beeswax. Catalog. Mail order.

Ladyslipper & Co

2848 Old Peachtree Road

Dacula, GA 30211

Wildflower essences. Catalog. Mail order.

M. J. Designs

972-304-2200

Essential and fragrant oils. Containers. Beeswax. Call for the location of the store nearest you.

Mid-Continent Agrimarketing

1465 N. Winchester

Olathe, KS 66061

800-547-1392

Bottles, jars, and other glass containers available in quantities as small as six. Catalog. Mail order.

Index

CREDITS

Breslich & Foss are grateful to the following individuals and institutions for permission to reproduce illustrations:
Tony Stone Images: p.75. Images Colour Library Ltd: p.7, p.14, p.24, p.60, p.76, p.101, p.102, p.110. Zefa Pictures: p.23, p.59, p.109.

Cover:

Background image: Image Bank.
Front cover, left to right: Tony Stone Images, Image Bank, Zefa, Tony Stone Images, Images Colour Library.

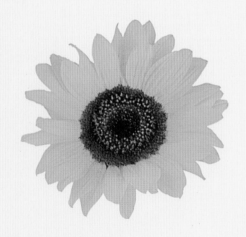